Penguin Books

Acupuncture for Everyone

Dr Ruth Lever qualified from St Mary's Hospital, London, with the degrees of M.B., B.S. Her career in orthodox medicine has included work in paediatrics, psychiatry and public health and she has an M.Sc. in social medicine from London University.

For four and a half years she was Medical Officer in Charge of Troops at a large Army depot and it was during this period that she started to study and practise various alternative therapies including acupuncture, hypnosis, healing and nutrition counselling. Since leaving Army practice, she has started writing on various aspects of orthodox and alternative medicine and has appeared regularly on the T V S programme *Problem Page*.

She is now in practice with her husband, who is a homoeopath.

RUTH LEVER

ACUPUNCTURE FOR EVERYONE

PENGUIN BOOKS

Penguin Books Ltd, Harmondsworth, Middlesex, England
Viking Penguin Inc., 40 West 23rd Street, New York, New York 10010, U.S.A.
Penguin Books Australia Ltd, Ringwood, Victoria, Australia
Penguin Books Canada Ltd, 2801 John Street, Markham, Ontario, Canada L3R 1B4
Penguin Books (N.Z.) Ltd, 182–190 Wairau Road, Auckland 10, New Zealand

First published by Penguin Books 1987

Made and printed in Great Britain by
Richard Clay Ltd, Bungay, Suffolk
Typeset in 11/13 Monophoto Plantin

CONTENTS

For Marie Ross

ACKNOWLEDGEMENTS

There have been so many things which have led up to my writing this book and I should like to thank all those people whose help and encouragement in the past have enabled it to come about: Dr Martin Woodhouse, Mrs Marie Ross, Michael Endacott, Anthony Baird, Jane Foulkes, the late Dr Jos. Leigh, Miss Miriam E. Shillito, Tom Dummer, Judith O'Hagen, Patricia Borwick, my husband, John, and my parents.

I would also like to thank Mr Roger Murray of Lewes, Sussex, for his permission to quote several of the case histories in Chapter Seven.

INTRODUCTION

Nowadays, as a result of the great surge of public interest in matters of health, one can hardly pick up a magazine or turn on the television without seeing something about one of the many complementary, or alternative, therapies that are becoming increasingly popular in the West. Some, such as homoeopathy, have been fairly well known for many years whereas others, such as acupuncture, have only just been 'discovered' by patients who are becoming dissatisfied with the drug-orientated therapies of twentieth-century orthodox medicine.

In Europe and North America, increasing numbers of people are trying acupuncture in an attempt to find relief from all manner of complaints. Like all therapies, orthodox or otherwise, it does not work for everyone, so while some patients will derive benefit and will recommend acupuncture to their friends, others will give up the treatment and go on to try something else.

However, among those people whose health improves after a course of acupuncture, there must be some who wonder just how much of the improvement was due to the treatment and how much was fortuitous – did it just happen that their illness took a turn for the better at the same time that they started going to the acupuncturist? Or could it have been mind over matter? Because, even to those who have experienced acupuncture, and very much more to those who haven't, it can seem a rather bizarre form of treatment. In the tradition of Western medicine, we are accustomed to having treatment directed at the part of the body that is malfunctioning – if you have a sprained ankle you strap it, if you have a boil you lance it and if you have an inflamed appendix you remove it. But acupuncture treats all ailments by sticking needles into the skin and, very often, it seems that the needles are put into areas of the body that appear to be totally unrelated to the illness from which the patient is suffering.

Once one has found a qualified acupuncturist, he will be able to explain some of the fundamentals and this will help to answer some of the questions in the patient's mind. But first, one has got to pluck up courage to make the appointment. Whenever one sees a cartoon about acupuncture, it always shows someone stuck full of needles, looking something like Custer's Last Stand. And this, together with a lack of knowledge about the subject, can make the prospect of going for treatment in the first place quite frightening. We see this even in Western medicine: a patient will tolerate treatment and investigations far more readily if he is told in advance what is being done and why. But it takes a brave patient, already somewhat intimidated by the fact of having things done to him, to speak up and ask, 'What exactly are you doing that for? And what do you intend to do next?' So the purpose of this book is to try to explain what the acupuncturist is doing and why.

Throughout this book doctors, acupuncturists and patients are referred to as 'he'. This does not, of course, imply that there are no women doctors, acupuncturists or patients, but is to prevent the reader from becoming irritated by a constant repetition of 'he or she'.

In order to understand the theory of acupuncture, one has to forget all the concepts of Western medicine that one has been brought up with. For not only is this theory couched in terms evolved in an alien (Chinese) culture but it is also far more esoteric than the flesh-and-bones theories of Western medicine. The latter treats the physical matter of the body. If its function has become disrupted it treats it with drugs – for example, giving anti-hypertensives to treat raised blood pressure. If a part has become seemingly irreparably diseased, or is doing the patient harm, it is surgically removed – for example, the removal of an inflamed appendix or an overactive thyroid gland. Or if the part has merely become distorted, it may be surgically repaired – for example, the repair of a prolapsed womb. And for parts of the body whose function is inadequate, there is a variety of therapies whose aim is to encourage the return of normal function by stimulating the affected part – for example, physiotherapy in the case of poorly functioning muscles and psychotherapy for mental problems.

Acupuncture, however, is a single therapy, using the insertion of needles into the skin to treat a variety of ailments which might be treated by Western doctors with drugs or surgery or stimulatory therapies. The reason why it is able to treat all ailments in the same way is because it sees them as stemming from the same cause – a disruption to the energy flow or vital force of the body. This vital force, of which much more will be said in Chapter Two, does not play a role in Western medicine. In Chinese medicine it is seen as the fundamental force which maintains the function of the body, therefore any disruption of its flow can cause malfunction and disease. So acupuncture treatment aims to restore balance to this energy flow which is said to run through a system of channels, or meridians, to supply the entire body. The location of a particular disease is determined by which part or parts of the body are supplied by the affected meridian. Stimulation of the meridian by the insertion of needles at various defined points along its length can restore the flow to normal and thus return the associated part to its normal function.

There are many ways in which these points may be stimulated that do not entail the use of needles. The word 'acupuncture' implies the use of needles since it is derived from two words: the Latin 'acu', meaning 'with a needle', and the English 'puncture' It is thus something of a misnomer (as well as being a word of Western origin describing an Oriental therapy) since it is not the actual piercing of the skin that is the important part of the treatment, but the stimulation of the points that lie along the meridians. Some practitioners, in fact, just refer to their practice as 'meridian therapy' although, to the public, this is even more obscure than the term 'acupuncture'.

Needles are, of course, the most commonly used method of stimulating the points. However, pressure may be used in a form of massage, or the points may be warmed (or even burned, as I shall mention in the next chapter, on the history of acupuncture). Lasers have also been used to stimulate the points and it is nowadays even possible to buy a 'do it yourself' acupuncture kit, complete with electrical stimulator with which to treat your own points. However, the latter is not to be recommended because, as will become clear, without a thorough training in the theory and practice of acupuncture, it is rather like buying a knife and an anatomy book and trying to take out your own appendix!

This is not, therefore, a teach yourself acupuncture book. What I will try to do is to demonstrate how an acupuncturist makes his diagnosis and how, in the light of this diagnosis, he treats his patient. The aim is to give the patient enough knowledge about the subject to make the step of actually going to an acupuncturist for the first time less intimidating. And it is to try to throw light on some of the mysteries that the therapist may not have time to explain during the treatment – such as why, if you go complaining of a headache, he may stick a needle in your foot!

Acupuncture originated, of course, in a culture quite different from our own and was only exported to the West comparatively late in its evolution. Its history, therefore, is a fundamental part of what it is today, and it is to its history that the next chapter is devoted.

CHAPTER ONE

A SHORT HISTORY

OF ACUPUNCTURE

Acupuncture is one of the oldest therapies known to man, having been in use for well over two thousand years. And although, from time to time, developments have occurred, the basic theory and practice are still much the same as when it was practised twenty centuries ago.

The fundamental theories of acupuncture are the same as those of Chinese medicine as a whole. In the West, all diagnoses made by doctors are based on our knowledge of anatomy, physiology, biochemistry and pathology. Once the patient has been diagnosed, the decision is made as to whether to treat him with drugs, surgery or other techniques. In the same way, acupuncture is one of the treatments that may be used when diagnoses are based on the ancient theories of Chinese medicine. As such, it may be used in conjunction with Chinese herbal medicine although, in the West, it is usually used alone.

The oldest known book on the theory of Chinese medicine is the *Nei Ching*, known in English as *The Yellow Emperor's Classic of Internal Medicine*. It is written in the form of a dialogue, the two participants being Huang Ti (the Yellow Emperor) and Ch'i Po, a Taoist teacher and physician. (In ancient times, the physicians were often, in addition, religious teachers. A not dissimilar state was found in the West, where monks were often highly skilled in herbal medicine.)

The Yellow Emperor is said to have lived in the twenty-seventh century B.C. In fact, there is dispute among scholars as to whether he even lived at all or whether he was just a mythical emperor – a legend perhaps based originally on a real person but, over the centuries, endowed with far more greatness than he actually warranted. It is rather like the arguments that take place in Britain as to whether there was really a King Arthur. However, even if the Yellow Emperor was a real person, it is highly unlikely that the *Nei Ching* can be attributed to him or that it dates from the time of his reign. In the twentieth century B.C., written Chinese was still in a fairly primitive form, known as archaic (or pre-historic) ideographs. The *Nei Ching* is an extremely profound work and it would have been impossible for much of it to have been expressed in this primitive script. It is generally agreed by scholars, therefore, that the *Nei Ching* was written during the so-called Warring States period – between 481 B.C. and 221 B.C. This, of course, still makes it a work of considerable antiquity.

However, although the *Nei Ching* is the oldest book on Chinese medicine that has come down to us, it was probably not the first book that was ever written on the subject for it is not written as a book that is introducing something new and original. In fact, by the time that it was written, somewhere between the fifth and the third centuries B.C., acupuncture was obviously widely understood and practised in China. The *Nei Ching* gives the reader no instruction whatsoever on the basic theory of acupuncture nor on the points and techniques to be used, and the topics it covers include the more esoteric aspects of acupuncture theory such as 'the transmission of the essence and the transformation of the life-giving principle' and 'the seasons as patterns of the viscera'. The Yellow Emperor asks the questions and these are then answered at length by Ch'i Po. Some of the questions are several pages long, and among the things that Ch'i Po is asked to explain are 'how it is possible that the twelve viscera send each other that which is precious and that which is worthless' and 'whether the brain and the marrow govern the viscera or whether it is the stomach that governs the viscera, or whether the viscera govern the six bowels'. The Yellow Emperor – real or mythical – obviously had a very good grasp of the basic theories of Chinese medicine!

Stories of great acupuncturists have also come down to us from two thousand years ago or more. Around the same time that the *Nei Ching* is thought to have been written, although somewhat after the time of the Yellow Emperor himself, there was a famous Chinese physician called Pien Chueh. His actual dates are unknown but, traditionally, he is said to have lived in the fourth century B.C., so it is possible that he may even have predated the *Nei Ching* by a hundred years or so. One story told about him says that Pien Chueh, who was, apparently, a wandering physician and teacher of medicine, was visiting the province of Kuo with some of his students, or apprentices. On reaching the town in which the king and his court resided, they saw many sacrifices being offered at the temples and arrangements being made for a funeral. Pien Chueh asked what was happening and was told that the prince of the province had fallen ill very suddenly and had lapsed into a coma from which the court physicians had been unable to rouse him. It seemed inevitable that he was going to die. Pien Chueh asked his informant whether he could arrange for him to be introduced at court, since he thought he might be able to prevent the prince from dying. Arrangements were made accordingly, and he was received by the king who willingly allowed him to examine the comatose prince.

After a thorough examination, Pien Chueh made a diagnosis based on his great knowledge of Chinese medicine. He then treated the prince, using acupuncture needles placed in his head, chest, arms and legs. Following this treatment, the prince rapidly regained consciousness. Pien Chueh continued to treat him and to monitor his progress for a further three weeks. In addition to acupuncture, he used heat treatment and herbal remedies. At the end of this period, the prince was fully restored to health. What happened to the court physicians the story does not tell, but it is possible that the king made arrangements for them to learn the basics of acupuncture!

When the story tells of Pien Chueh using heat to treat his patient, it may be referring to moxibustion, a therapy that is still very much in use today. Moxibustion is a method of stimulating the acupuncture points by heat. Its name derives from the herb that is burned to supply the heat, and which is known as moxa. Nowadays it is usual to attach a small wad of moxa to the end of an acupuncture needle which has already been inserted into the patient, so that, when it is lit, the heat travels down the needle and into the point, without running the risk of burning the patient. Originally it was the custom to put the moxa directly onto the patient's skin or on a slice of ginger placed over the relevant acupuncture point, and this method is still used by some practitioners. Some ancient texts have been found that mention the use of moxa but do not mention acupuncture and it is therefore possible that the practice of moxibustion predates that of acupuncture. However, these particular texts were found in a tomb that dates back to the Han dynasty (206 B.C.–A.D. 220), a period when, as we know from other sources, acupuncture was already widely used. But, of course, the texts themselves may be copies of others that were considerably older.

The moxa that is used today comes in a roll and is made of dried leaves which, when burned, smell not unlike cannabis – or so I have been told by a younger patient who informed me that my consulting room smelled like a pop festival! Moxa has the ability to burn slowly and steadily (again, not unlike cannabis or, of course, that other dried leaf of ill repute, tobacco). It has been in use for many centuries but the healing ability of warmth applied to the acupuncture points was probably known long before the burning properties of moxa leaves were discovered. It is probable that, originally, twigs and grass were used to produce a similar effect. It is known from the records that various other substances, such as charcoal, bamboo and sulphur, have all been used in the past.

Moxa is used primarily in the treatment of diseases which have been caused by cold or damp (this will be discussed in depth in Chapter Four). And although it was, and still is, often found to be useful in its homeland of China, it was used to a far greater extent in Japan. Being made up of islands, Japan tends to have a far more humid climate than the great expanse of China and therefore the incidence of disease which was due to damp was much greater. It is therefore appropriate that the name by which this treatment is known in the West – moxa – should, in fact, be Japanese in origin, derived from two words which mean 'burning herb'. The Chinese name for moxa is chiu, which means to cauterize or blister.

It has been suggested that it might have been through acupuncture points becoming accidentally burned that their therapeutic value was originally discovered. Acupuncture is such an ancient therapy that its origins are completely unknown. Strangely, in view of the fact that Chinese culture has many ancient legends and folk heroes, there is not even, as far as I know, any legend explaining how it originated. The burns theory is one of several that have been put forward. It suggests that in the days when people huddled round fires which served the dual purpose of keeping them warm and cooking their food, it was more than likely that they would frequently be burned by sparks flying out from the fire. If the spark landed on and the burn occurred on an appropriate acupuncture point, it might be that people would be 'miraculously' cured of various illnesses which had been troubling them. After a period of time, when this had happened on a number of occasions and to a number of people, they might have started to realize that there was something about these particular points on the body which had healing properties. In some patients, stimulation of a single point will cause a sensation to run along the meridian on which it lies. In other patients, one can sometimes see a flush spreading along the line of the meridian. Based on this, these early Chinese could have started to work out a system of lines which joined the points together – the predecessors of the meridians that we know today. And, of course, it would appear to them that the way in which to use these points therapeutically was to burn them, since it was through burning that the effects seemed to arise. This, then, ties in with the point made earlier that moxa treatment of the acupuncture points may well have developed before acupuncture itself was thought of.

Another theory concerning the origin of acupuncture is that, in the days when there was constant warring between neighbouring tribes, men who were wounded in battle may have found that injuries inflicted in certain spots had a therapeutic effect on various diseases from which they were suffering. This is a theory much loved by cartoonists who depict men run through with spears or stuck full of arrows saying things such as 'That's done wonders for my hay fever'. However, what still remains a mystery is why, when men were huddled round fires and involved in battles all over the world, it was only the Chinese who developed the idea of the meridians and treatment by acupuncture.

Once the points had been discovered, the next stage was to experiment with methods of stimulating them. The earliest acupuncture tools seem to have been sharp pieces of stone or flint, which were known as bian stones. Their use would have been limited, because of their size and shape, and they were probably used just to scratch, or perhaps prick, the points on the meridians. Sharp pieces of pottery were also used. The next instruments to be developed were somewhat more versatile and were made from sharpened bones and bamboo, which could be formed into a more needle-like shape. However, it was not until the discoveries concerning the smelting of metal had been made that it was possible to manufacture true needles that could actually be inserted through the patient's skin and into the layers below.

The earliest needles were made from various types of metals as they became available – iron, bronze, silver and even gold. Since metal was so much more versatile than the stones, bones and bamboo which had previously been used, it was possible to develop different shapes of needle which could then be used for different techniques. These may originally have been made by chance, since, presumably, the earliest metal-smithing was a fairly crude affair and one could not expect to get identical needles every time. However, the early acupuncture practitioners, presented with these varying shapes, may have realized that by using different shapes of needle they could produce different effects and, therefore, as the quality of the smithing improved, they would have ordered the specific shapes that they found most useful.

When the *Nei Ching* was written, nearly 2500 years ago, nine types of needle were already in common use, and these were not at all unlike the variety of needles that are still used today. There were fine needles which, as now, were used for the majority of straightforward treatments. There were arrowhead needles which were used when it was only necessary to prick the point, rather than to insert a needle. To induce slight bleeding at a point, three-sided needles were available. Needles with a triangular tip terminating in a sharp point are still used today when bleeding is required. Blunt or round-ended needles were used when points needed pressure or massaging and scalpel-like needles were used for incising boils and abscesses. Larger, heavier needles were available for treatments that necessitated a needle being inserted into a joint. Extra-long needles were used when the most receptive part of the acupuncture point lay well below the skin surface in an area of thick muscle or fat. Today, needles up to three inches long are used in areas such as the buttocks but even these are considerably shorter than some which are said to have been used by the early acupuncturists.

Silver and gold acupuncture needles have been found in the tomb of Prince Liu Sheng who lived and died some time during the period of the Western Han dynasty (206 B.C.–A.D. 24). It would seem, from their inclusion in the burial goods, that the people of the period thought that, even in heaven, one's health might need attention!

Stainless steel was first developed in the early years of the twentieth century and proved itself to be invaluable in medical treatment around the world. Nowadays it is used to make not only the surgical instruments and hypodermic needles employed in orthodox medicine but also the majority of needles used in acupuncture practice. Its great advantage is that it can be easily sterilized and will not rust. Before its development, silver and gold acupuncture needles were probably more widely used than they are today because these two metals are relatively inert and less likely to cause unwanted reactions when inserted into patients. There may also have been other reasons for their popularity: it was thought that gold needles had, of themselves, a stimulating effect (this was also said to be true of the other yellow metal, copper) while silver and other white metal needles had a calming effect. Today, needles made of precious metals have definite disadvantages in that they are very much more expensive than stainless steel and are too valuable to be thrown away when they become blunt, and so have to be resharpened. However, some practitioners are still sufficiently convinced of their intrinsic therapeutic effects to go on using them. A letter was published recently in the *American Journal of Acupuncture* (vol. 13, no. 4, December 1985) from a doctor in Spain who has found that he obtains the best results when treating pain by using gold needles for patients whose pain is made worse by movement or patients with pain that is due to inflammation or disuse, and silver needles when the pain is due to over-use of the part concerned.

A number of modern practitioners, especially those who trained in China, continue the ancient Chinese practice of using herbal medicine and acupuncture together in the treatment of their patients. This form of herbal medicine differs from that used in the West in that it is based on the same fundamental theories of body function and energy flow as acupuncture. Therefore in China it was natural that the two should be taught together, rather as both general medicine and surgery are taught to Western medical students.

The first state-sponsored medical school in China, which taught all aspects of Chinese medicine, was founded in A.D. 443 but it was closed again within ten years. Student physicians had to revert to the traditional method of learning which was by apprenticeship to an experienced physician. In A.D. 581, under the Sui dynasty, an Imperial Medical Academy was founded. However, it was under the following Tang dynasty (A.D. 618–906) that medical education really started to develop. In A.D. 624 the Academy was greatly enlarged and departments were set up to teach pharmacology, acupuncture, internal medicine, massage, and also Buddhist and Taoist incantation which, at that time, were thought to be essential knowledge for a physician. For the first time, it became possible to study acupuncture and moxibustion as a separate discipline from herbal medicine.

The length of time that it took to train to become a physician was somewhat longer than that taken by Western medical students today. Before a student could specialize in any one aspect of medicine, he had to take a general basic course. When he had passed this, he was allowed to go on to study internal medicine, which took a further seven years of study, or surgery, which took five years, or paediatrics, which also took five years. Less time was required to study more limited subjects, such as diseases of the ear, nose and throat.

Like medical schools today, the Imperial Medical Academy taught from standard textbooks. The *Nei Ching* was, of course, one. Another was Huang-Pu Mi's *Chia I Ching* (*The Classic of Acupuncture Fundamentals*) which was written in the third century A.D. and is the oldest known book of its kind, being devoted entirely to acupuncture and moxibustion. Many later books used the *Chia I Ching* as a source book and it played an important role in the development of acupuncture in Japan and Korea. A third standard text in use at the Imperial Medical Academy was Wang Su-Ho's *Mai Ching* (*The Classic of the Pulse*).

Pulse-taking is a much more exact and detailed science in Chinese medicine than it is in Western medicine and plays a far more important role in diagnosis. It may take a student many years to become an expert in interpreting the pulse fully. And because not just acupuncture but all forms of traditional Chinese medicine are based on the same theories of the causation of disease, pulse diagnosis is fundamental to them all. Wang Su-Ho's *Classic of the Pulse* was not expounding a newly developed science but was a compilation of ancient diagnostic techniques which had grown up alongside Chinese medicine as it developed. Other books, published long before Wang Su-Ho's, had mentioned pulse diagnosis, including, of course, the *Nei Ching* which gives some quite detailed descriptions as to the quality of the pulse in different disease states. The great acupuncturist Pien Chueh, whom we have already met in the story of his treatment of the comatose prince of Kuo, is known to have used pulse diagnosis. It may, of course, have been his skill as a diagnostician, rather than his choice of treatment, that enabled him to treat the prince successfully, when the court physicians had failed.

Pien Chueh is said to have been the first physician to use together the four basic techniques of Chinese diagnosis. The first of these techniques was observation, in which the physician took note of his patient's complexion, colour, skin and tongue in much the same way that a Western physician would do today, although, of course, his findings would be interpreted differently, according to traditional Chinese theory. The tongue, like the pulse, can tell a traditionally trained Chinese physician far more than it can reveal in Western medicine and is an important method of diagnosis. (More will be said about these methods in Chapter Five.) The physician would also observe his patient's expression, as this too might aid the diagnosis. The second technique, or group of techniques, used by Pien Chueh was listening and smelling. He would listen to the quality of the patient's speech – whether it was normal, slurred, high pitched and so on – and to the sound of his breathing, although without the benefit of that modern Western tool, the stethoscope. He would smell the patient's body odours – probably more important in a society where hot and cold running water was unknown and baths were probably taken infrequently. However, this technique is still used by some acupuncture practitioners and is even occasionally of use in Western practice today, where the smell of acetone on a patient's breath is accepted as a clear indication that he is a diabetic whose condition is getting out of control. The third technique in Pien Chueh's list was questioning which, of course, plays a very important part in all forms of medicine – orthodox, Chinese and other complementary therapies. And finally, he would use pulse diagnosis.

The Classic of the Pulse was exported to Japan and Korea in the sixth century A.D. Chinese medicine had reached both countries several centuries earlier and techniques of pulse diagnosis were rapidly assimilated into the medical practice of both countries. The *Chu Ping Yuan Hou Lun* (*A Discourse on the Causes and Symptoms of All Illnesses*), published only a few years later in A.D. 610, was also to become extremely influential in the development of Japanese and Korean medicine. Its grandiose title was, perhaps, justified since it stretched to fifty volumes and was a compilation of virtually all of the medical knowledge of the time. Its editor was Chao Yuan Fang, a physician at the Imperial court.

As Chinese medicine developed during the Tang dynasty, its fame spread and physicians from other nations came to China to learn new techniques. Arabian physicians came to learn the art of pulse diagnosis and to study infectious diseases. *The Classic of the Pulse* was actually exported to the Middle East some time in the eleventh century and, by the mid-fourteenth century, it had been translated into Turkish. The great Persian physician, Abu-Ali al-Husain ibn Abdullah ibn Sina, better known as Avicenna (980–1037), wrote an immense work in Arabic called *Al-Qanun fi'l-Tibb* (*The Canon of Medicine*) in which he discussed the medical achievements of the great Greek physicians and described medical techniques that had been written about in other Arabic works. To this he added information about the techniques that he himself had developed during his own years of practice, based on what he had learned from reading and had been taught during his travels. He wrote about the use of pulse diagnosis and recorded twenty-four different types of pulse of which he was aware.

It was mainly due to the patronage of the nobility and the Emperors that acupuncture and moxibustion became very popular in China during the Sung dynasty (960–1279). Despite this, and despite the fact that acupuncture and the diagnostic techniques of Chinese medicine were now becoming familiar in other parts of Asia and in the Middle East, there was a feeling at the Chinese Imperial court that over the years inaccuracies had arisen in the practice of this therapy. Many of the early books on acupuncture had been lost and many of the standard reference books were compilations into which errors might have crept. In the eleventh century, Wang Wei-I, who was the court physician to two of the Emperors of the Northern Sung dynasty, Chen-Tsung (997–1022) and Jen-Tsung (1022–1063), was instructed to investigate the validity of the system of acupuncture that was currently being practised and to carry out what would be the first major revision of acupuncture theory.

Wang Wei-I embarked on a mammoth research programme. He investigated all the acupuncture points that were currently being used and verified their locations. He also studied each point in turn and confirmed to what depth each should be punctured by the needle in order to produce an effect. Finally, he identified the effects that might be produced by the puncture of each point. He published his findings in a book entitled *The New Illustrated Manual on the Points for Acupuncture*.

Wang Wei-I's exact dates are unknown and he may well have died before 1034, which was the year in which his Imperial patron, Emperor Jen-Tsung, was taken ill. The Emperor, who was an orthodox Confucian and a patron of scholars, was twenty-two years old at the time and had been attended by the Imperial physicians who, using methods other than acupuncture, had been unable to cure him. Eventually he was successfully treated with acupuncture by a highly skilled acupuncturist named Xu Xi. However, the courtiers attending the Emperor nearly forbade the treatment to take place, since Xu Xi, having examined the Emperor, let it be known that he proposed to insert acupuncture needles into his chest, just below the level of his heart. On hearing this, the courtiers were horrified and said that on no account must the treatment take place because, far from curing the Emperor, it would kill him. However, Xu Xi assured them that the treatment was quite safe and offered to demonstrate the technique on someone whose death, if it occurred, would be less of a disaster. This proposition was acceptable to the courtiers, who decided that he could demonstrate on the court eunuchs who, presumably, were expendable. Xu Xi inserted his needles into the eunuchs at the point that he had described and the courtiers were amazed and relieved to find that he had spoken the truth and that the eunuchs were unharmed. (No doubt the eunuchs were even more relieved!) Xu Xi was therefore allowed to return to the Emperor's presence and treat him in the manner that he had demonstrated. Fortunately for both Xu Xi and the Emperor, the latter made a rapid recovery following this. Everyone at court was so impressed by this demonstration of skill that Xu Xi was appointed medical officer of the Imperial Medical Academy.

Although it seems that the earlier court physicians attendant on Jen-Tsung were not particularly adept at acupuncture, Wang Wei-I, who served both him and the Emperor Chen-Tsung, is still remembered for the contribution he made to both the treatment itself and its teaching. He had a model of a man cast in bronze, the surface of which was punctured with holes, accurately placed at the positions of all the acupuncture points. This was, of course, based on all the research that he had undertaken when compiling his *New Illustrated Manual on the Points for Acupuncture*. Wang Wei-I's bronze men became a valuable teaching aid for students of acupuncture and were used in examinations held at the Imperial Medical Academy to test their knowledge. Before the examination, the model was covered with a thick layer of wax which was allowed to set so that the holes at the position of the acupuncture points could not be seen. The hollow interior of the model was then filled with water. The student who was sitting the exam was questioned about a case and was asked how he would treat it using acupuncture. Having said which points he would use and why, he was then asked to locate them on the model and was told to insert a needle into each of them, through the wax. If he located the points accurately, the needles would go through the wax and into the holes below so that, when the needles were removed, water would flow from the holes.

In the mid-sixteenth century, five hundred years after Wang Wei-I cast his first bronze model, his idea was developed by an acupuncturist named Kao Wu. Wang Wei-I's figures had all been of men but Kao Wu thought it important to demonstrate that the location of acupuncture points differed according to the sex and the age of the patient. He therefore had bronze figures cast of women and children, which could be used in the same way as Wang Wei-I's male figures.

Kao Wu believed that many errors had arisen in acupuncture practice since Wang Wei-I carried out his great investigation and he set himself the task of rectifying this. He wrote two important books on the subject, the first of which was called *Essentials of Acupuncture and Moxibustion*. This was a summary of earlier major acupuncture works and was intended as a guide for students of acupuncture who were just embarking on their course of studies. His other great work, entitled *Eminent Acupuncture*, was for more advanced students and practitioners already in practice and it gave detailed information about the meridians and the points and how they should be used in the treatment of a variety of diseases.

Like Kao Wu's *Essentials of Acupuncture and Moxibustion*, many of the 'new' acupuncture books that were being written around this time were simply revisions and summaries of the works of earlier authors. In 1601, however, the acupuncturist Yang Jizhou published a book entitled *A Compendium of Acupuncture and Moxibustion*. In this, not only did he summarize what had been written about acupuncture in previous centuries, but he also included much information that was based on the results of his own research and experience. Being an 'original', this book was a great success both in China and in other countries in Asia to which the practice of acupuncture had spread.

By this time, acupuncture and traditional Chinese medicine had spread far beyond the borders of China and in some countries, such as Japan and Korea, were the accepted form of medical treatment. Chinese medicine was first introduced into these two countries many centuries before, during the Chin dynasty (249–206 B.C.), but it was with the spread of Buddhism that it really began to gain popularity. Buddhism, which originated in India in the sixth century B.C., reached China some time around the middle of the first century A.D. There it developed in tradition and practice and, in the second half of the fourth century, was introduced into Korea. Some two hundred years later it spread to Japan, where the school of Zen Buddhism developed which is still widely practised today. Although the religion was not an immediate success among the Japanese people, the Regent Shotoku Taishi (593–622) was converted and began to encourage Buddhist monks to come to Japan from China.

In China Buddhist monks often studied Chinese medicine and acupuncture, and during the Sui (A.D. 589–618) and Tang (A.D. 618–906) dynasties many of these physician-monks came to Japan. While they were there, they taught the Japanese whatever they wished to learn – not just Buddhist doctrine but also the fundamentals of Chinese medicine.

All the early Buddhist texts had been written in Pali but, with the spread of the religion, more scriptures had been written in Sanskrit and in Chinese and earlier works had been translated. However, it took time before translations could be made for a newly converted country and all the texts being used by the monks who went to Japan were in Chinese. If the Japanese converts wanted to read the original scriptures and not just hear about them from the monks (who, no doubt, were putting their own interpretation onto them), they would have to learn to read Chinese. And this is what many of them did. Of course, having become proficient in Chinese, they could then read not only the scriptures but also all the texts from which the monks had been teaching them the essentials of medicine and acupuncture. Young Japanese men started to go to China to learn the language and, during the seventh century, many made the trip and came back with not just a knowledge of Chinese but of Chinese medicine as well.

Once enough Japanese physicians were fluent in the Chinese language, translations could be made of the major Chinese medical texts so that they would be available to all. The *Nei Ching* was one of the first to be translated and, by the beginning of the eighth century, was being used as one of the standard textbooks for Japanese medical students. Large numbers of Chinese medical books were brought to Japan in the mid-eighth century by a man named Chien-Chen who was both a physician and a philanthropist. He established a charity clinic in Japan for the treatment of the

poor and, centuries later, his memory was still being vener-
ated in Japanese temples as a result of his work with the sick
and needy.

Chinese medicine remained popular in Japan until the
sixteenth century when it became overshadowed by influences from the West. This was the period of the great
trading companies with ships being sent from Europe to
build up markets and find suppliers of luxuries in far-flung
places around the world. The Portuguese, who were ardent
believers in the superiority of Roman Catholicism over all
other, 'pagan' religions, sent ships to the Far East with more
in view than mere trading. Initially, the reception they
received was hostile since it was discovered that they were
only prepared to trade with people whom they could not
vanquish. Weaker communities ran the risk of being over-
run and massacred. However, having been allowed access
to only one town in the whole of China (and that being one
with which they had to trade), the second wave of this
Portuguese 'invasion' was somewhat gentler, consisting of
a number of missionaries who were able to gain a foothold
in both China and Japan. Like the Buddhist monks who
had come to Japan in the sixth century, these missionaries
had some knowledge of medicine although this, of course,
was the comparatively primitive medicine being practised
in Europe at the time. However, because it was new and
different, or perhaps because of the forceful personalities of
those who brought it to the East, it usurped the practice of
traditional Chinese medicine in Japan.

Over the next three centuries, acupuncture and Chinese
medicine played second fiddle to Western medicine in
Japan, although their practice continued. In 1884 an
attempt was made to wipe them out completely when an
edict prohibiting the teaching of acupuncture and herbal
medicine anywhere in the country was issued, to coincide
with the founding of the medical faculty of Tokyo univer-

sity. However, not even this could stop people from prac-
tising the therapies that they believed in and, up to the
present day, traditional medicine and acupuncture have
continued to be used alongside Western techniques.

Surprisingly, in 1822, sixty-two years before the teaching of acupuncture and Chinese medicine was prohibited in
Japan, their use was banned in their homeland, China, by
the Ch'ing dynasty Emperor Tao Kuang. The subjects
were removed from the syllabus at the Imperial Medical
Academy but, as was to happen later in Japan, their use
could not be stopped, since the people who had practised
them for many centuries were aware of their value and
would not give them up.

In 1912 the Imperial dynasty was overthrown and replaced by the radical Kuomintang party who ruled China
until the end of the Second World War when they, in turn,
were ousted by the Communists. The Communists, aware
of the people's views concerning acupuncture and traditional Chinese medicine, removed the prohibitions on their
use. Indeed, acupuncture was actively encouraged and
allowed to flourish. Many of the ancient Chinese medical
books that had been used over the centuries as standard
texts were reprinted and many new books were written.
Colleges specializing in the teaching of traditional Chinese
medicine were set up, all with separate departments of acupuncture. Research institutes were founded for the investigation of acupuncture and the furtherance of its practice
and in the existing medical schools which, since the ban of
1822, had taught nothing but Western medicine, acupuncture found its way onto the curriculum. China now has
many medical schools and, since 1949, acupuncture has
been taught in all of them, alongside Western medicine, in
an integrated course.

Acupuncture remains a popular therapy in a number of
Asian countries. In Vietnam, where it was introduced during

the Han dynasty (206 B.C.–A.D. 220), a system has grown up in recent years whereby acupuncture and traditional herbal medicine are used for everyday ills, but patients who are admitted to hospital are treated with Western techniques.

It is, perhaps, surprising that Western medicine which, until around the turn of this century was a fairly crude discipline with little to offer in the way of curative techniques, should have so easily superseded the practice of the far more sophisticated Chinese medicine and acupuncture in the Far East, particularly in Japan and China. Maybe it says something about the willingness of the Chinese and Japanese to accept'new ideas, compared with Westerners. Because, although acupuncture was introduced into Europe during the seventeenth century, at roughly the same time that Western medicine was having such an impact in the East, it did not attain popularity among Westerners until the second half of the twentieth century. This may be due to the fact that when Western medicine was introduced to the East, it was still in its infancy and thus the Chinese and Japanese could learn about its development gradually, whereas acupuncture was already a highly developed therapy, and, for the Western mind, very hard to understand, by the time that it was introduced into Europe.

Interest in acupuncture really only developed in the West when it was realized that it could be used in place of an anaesthetic for controlling pain during operations. The use of acupuncture to relieve pain caused by disease had, of course, been known for centuries in the countries where it was practised. However, surgery only started to be used on a large scale at the end of the last century and it was only in 1958 that Chinese doctors started to use acupuncture to control post-operative pain. The results they obtained were so good that they decided to see whether it was possible to control the pain of a minor operation – tonsillectomy was the first to be tried – without having to use any other form of anaesthesia. Again, the results were excellent and they began to use acupuncture for other minor operations such as tooth extractions and the repair of hernias. Although they found that not all patients treated with acupuncture would develop a sufficient degree of anaesthesia to allow it to be used as the sole method of pain control during an operation, many patients were able to tolerate surgery without any other method of anaesthesia being required. Nowadays, even major operations are performed regularly in China's hospitals using only acupuncture to stop the pain. The advantages of this are, of course, enormous, since the risks and unpleasant side effects associated with drug-induced anaesthesia are avoided.

Most people in the West probably first became aware of acupuncture when its use as an anaesthetic was discussed in the medical journals and in the popular press. But it was first introduced into Europe as long ago as the seventeenth century by individuals who had travelled to China under the auspices of the great trading companies. One of the first countries to show an interest in acupuncture was France and one of the earliest books to be written on acupuncture by a European was by the Frenchman Placide Harvieu (1671–1746). It was splendidly entitled *The Secrets of Chinese Medicine, and the Perfect Knowledge of the Pulse, Brought from China by a Respected Frenchman*. Soon afterwards, another book on acupuncture was published in France written by the Reverend Father Cleyer but he, presumably, was not intending to appeal to a wide audience, since he wrote it in Latin!

Another Frenchman was probably the first European actually to practise acupuncture, Dr Louis-Joseph Berlioz (1776–1848). Sadly, his pioneering work is scarcely remembered and the name of Berlioz is associated in most people's minds only with his famous son, the composer Hector

Berlioz. However, Dr Berlioz left behind him a book, *Memoirs on Chronic Complaints*, which he had had published in 1816 and in which he devoted a chapter to the practice of acupuncture.

A section on acupuncture was also included in a book entitled *Chinese Medicine*, which was published in 1863 by P. Dabry who, at the time that he wrote it, was the French consul in China. However, despite the fact that Frenchmen were interested enough in acupuncture to continue to investigate it and write about it, few of them actually practised the therapy themselves.

During the early nineteenth century, some references to acupuncture began to creep into English medical literature, but the main interest in the subject remained on the continent. In the early years of the twentieth century, Georges Soulie de Morant, who was resident in China as the representative of a French bank, decided to study acupuncture himself and, at the end of his studies, he was awarded the title of Master Physician. He remained in China for twenty years, going on to become the French consul and, during this time, he translated into French several works on Chinese medicine, as well as writing two books of his own. Of these, *The Synopsis of the True Chinese Acupuncture* was published in 1934 and *Acupuncture* was published in two volumes in 1939.

A modern development of acupuncture for which France has been mainly responsible is ear acupuncture or auriculotherapy. Points have been found in the ear which are associated with individual parts of the body – for example, a lung point, a stomach point, a knee point and so on – and the patient is treated by having needles inserted into the points relating to the location of his disease. This method was developed by Dr Nogier who published *A Treatise of Auriculotherapy* in 1972.

Acupuncture has been in use in England since the 1950s.

In 1957, Dr Louis Moss, a London GP, published a paper in the *Lancet* in which he reported the results of the treatment of some 2000 patients who were suffering from arthritis. Dr Moss had found that treatment of certain 'trigger points' gave these patients permanent relief from pain and he pointed out that these points tallied well with the position of certain acupuncture points.

Interest was now aroused in some members of the British medical profession and, the following year, a group of doctors visited Germany where acupuncture had been practised in a small way for many years. The theory of acupuncture had originally been introduced into Germany at the end of the seventeenth century by Engelbert Kaempfer, a naturalist and traveller, who devoted two chapters of his *History of Japan* to the subject. In 1906, at a time when the establishment of a Chinese medicine research institute in Germany was sparking off the publication of many new books on traditional Chinese medicine and acupuncture in the German language, Kaempfer's book had been translated into English but had had little impact on the British doctors of the day.

Recent interest in acupuncture in the West, however, stems from President Nixon's visit to China which seemed to stimulate Western interest in all aspects of the country and its culture. Of course, the Chinese people who had, from the early nineteenth century, settled in the United States and Canada continued to follow their own customs and to practise traditional Chinese medicine. But the very fact that the Chinese remained within their own Chinatowns prevented the practice of acupuncture from spreading to the rest of the population. But though although few people outside the Chinese communities had experience of acupuncture, and probably none practised the therapy, there was some small interest in the subject and a few books were published, such as *The Chinese Way of Medicine* by

Edward Hume in 1940, and a partial translation of the *Nei Ching* by Ilza Veith in 1949. Although Dr Veith's skill in the Chinese language enabled her to produce a readable and informative translation of this very difficult work, it is quite clear that she had had no personal experience of acupuncture when she set to work on the book. For, in the introduction, she writes, 'even the practice of acupuncture and moxibustion has survived, despite the fact that these treatments must be exceedingly painful to the patient' – clear indication that she had never even seen a patient being treated with acupuncture. In fact, in the preface to the revised 1965 edition of the book, she writes, 'at the time of the ... publication of this work, the subject of my study seemed to be entirely esoteric'.

In the last few years, acupuncture has grown enormously in popularity in the West. In Britain there are now a number of colleges which teach traditional Chinese medicine and acupuncture and there is no shortage of patients wishing to see their graduate practitioners.

CHAPTER TWO

FUNDAMENTAL PRINCIPLES

Acupuncture, as it has been used over the centuries by the Chinese, can truly be described as a holistic therapy. Many people, however, have become confused as to what is actually meant by the word 'holistic', which has been bandied around in recent years, particularly when complementary (non-orthodox) therapies are under discussion. Indeed, it seems that some people who have incorporated it into their vocabularies really have no clear idea of what it means. Therefore, before extolling the virtues of acupuncture as a holistic therapy, it is, I think, necessary to say a little about holism itself.

Holism

The word 'holism' seems to have been coined in the 1920s by Jan Smuts to mean, in the words of the Oxford English Dictionary, 'the tendency in nature to produce wholes from the ordered grouping of units'. Sometimes one sees it spelled 'wholism' but, since Smuts derived it from the Greek word 'holos' (meaning whole) and not from the English word 'whole' it should be spelled without a 'w'. Thus 'holistic' means encompassing the whole and, in terms of medicine, means treating the patient as a whole. Some people, however, use the word as synonymous with 'complementary' or 'alternative' when speaking about medical therapies. But, of course, this usage is incorrect for, although most alternative therapies are holistic when properly used, it is still perfectly possible to use them in a non-holistic way.

In recent years, the idea of holism has crept into the orthodox medical world and medical practitioners in the United
States and in Britain have formed their own holistic medical
associations. Much of holism resides in the attitude of the
therapist to his patient and thus, in the same way that it is
possible for complementary therapies to be practised in a
non-holistic way, it is perfectly possible, and commendable,
for an orthodox practitioner to practise holistically by taking
account of all his patient's problems and relating them to the
patient as a whole. Indeed, this was the virtue of the old-
fashioned family doctor, compared with today's overworked
health centre general practitioner. The family doctor knew
each of his patients individually, he knew their parents, their
husbands or wives, and their children, since all of them
would have been his patients too. He knew where his
patients worked, the sort of food that they could afford and
the kind of housing they lived in. He was a part of the com-
munity – he lived in the same town or village as his patients
and got to know them socially. When he made a house call to
visit one patient, he would probably be afforded a chance to
speak to other members of the family, many of whom would
be living locally. It was therefore a great deal easier for him
to see the patient as a whole than it is for a GP today, whose
patients often live in isolated units remote from the rest of
their family, whose backgrounds and places of work he does
not know and who may have only become his patients in
adult life, with their previous medical notes written in a
totally indecipherable hand.

Sadly, the trend towards holism within the medical profession, although admirable, will not be easy to follow
through for, with today's larger and more mobile popula-
tions, we will never be able to return to the old family doctor days. A further problem is that, no matter how
holistically inclined the practitioner, orthodox medicine *per
se* is not a holistic therapy, since the majority of treatments

now available are based on the use of drugs and of surgery. Surgery, of course, cannot be holistic – it is based on the principle that if a part of the patient is diseased, that part is removed. Drug therapy can be starkly contrasted with one of the complementary therapies, homoeopathy, in which, in order to work to the best advantage, the remedy given must relate to all aspects of the patient and not just the symptoms of which he is complaining. Modern drugs, on the other hand, are formulated to have a specific action on only one or two particular complaints. Thus we have anti-arthritic drugs, hypotensive and cardioprotective drugs (to bring down the blood pressure and protect the heart), tranquillizers and sleeping pills. And this is why people with several complaints find themselves having to take a number of different tablets to control them. If a patient is suffering from bronchitis, arthritis and bad eyesight, a holistic therapy used correctly may well produce an improvement in all three complaints, since its action is to raise the level of health of the whole patient, allowing his body to 'fight back' against the conditions that are troubling him. However, there is no way that an orthodox practitioner can prescribe a single medication that will do this, much as he might like to; nor has any orthodox drug been found that can raise the patient's entire level of health. The old-fashioned tonics were supposed to do this but, of course, they contained only stimulants, such as strychnine, and iron to cure any iron-deficiency anaemia which might happen to be contributing to the patient's malaise. But this sort of treatment is quite possible for a truly holistic therapy.

The point about a holistic therapy is that it does not treat a single symptom, nor even a disease. It treats a patient. And each patient is an individual, unlike any other. Although they may not treat them as such, orthodox doctors are also well aware of this. The controlled trials that are used in orthodox medicine to compare two forms of treatment, or to try to establish the efficacy of a new treatment, involve using two comparable groups of patients. And it is not always easy to find enough 'matched' patients even when the matching criteria are as basic as age, sex and the length of time that the patient has been ill. Think how much harder it would be to match patients if one also included things such as weight, temperament, marital status, number of children, job, standard of education, financial status, housing and so on. And yet these are all things which contribute to that patient being the person that he is.

So when one is using a holistic therapy, every patient is treated individually, because what may relieve the symptoms of one may have no effect at all on another who, in orthodox terms, appears to have the same complaint. Even in Western medicine, it is acknowledged that patients react differently to different drugs. Not all patients with arthritis, for example, can be treated with the same preparation; some will find it helpful but others will show little response or will develop side effects whose severity outweighs the relief obtained from taking the drug. And this is one reason why a large number of drugs may be available for the treatment of a single condition. Most doctors have their favourite drugs for common conditions – those which seem to them to be most effective and which they will always use as their first choice. But trying to find the right medication for a patient always has something of a hit-and-miss aspect about it, simply because one can never tell in advance exactly how this patient, as opposed to the last patient or the next one, will respond to a particular drug.

In acupuncture, however, the system of diagnosis is geared to finding an individual tailor-made treatment for an individual patient. In Western medicine, a diagnosis – and therefore the treatment of the patient on whom the diagnosis is made – is based on determining which particular organ or part is malfunctioning. The diagnosis is made in terms relating to that part, such as heart attack, gall bladder disease, kidney stones, slipped disc, varicose veins and so on. In other words, the diagnosis usually given is a description of the end result of the disease process. It is not related to the causative factors. This is not to say that orthodox medicine is not interested in preventive medicine, but the emphasis in disease remains firmly on the disease process and its end result.

Prevention, as well as diagnosis, can be undertaken on various levels. For instance, the prevention of infection can be done on three levels: the first is to give the patient a prophylactic antibiotic so that, if his system is invaded by bacteria, the antibiotic will kill them and he will not become ill; the second is to examine the environment, find where the bacteria are coming from, and eradicate them (this is the level at which most orthodox prevention works); the third level is to look at the patient and treat him, as a whole, so that his own natural defences are strong enough to resist any attack that may occur. This is the holistic idea of raising the level of health of the patient.

This, then, is the basis on which patients are treated by acupuncture. The diagnosis is concerned with how the energies of the body are malfunctioning rather than with the manifestations of disease which that malfunction has caused. The area in which the disease appears (such as the heart, gall bladder or kidney) is merely an indication of how the body has been affected by the disruption of its energies. In other words, heart disease does not mean that there is a problem heart in an otherwise healthy body nor even that the heart itself needs to be treated. What it does mean is that the patient's vital energies have become disrupted in such a way that it has manifested as disease of the heart. The disease manifestation is simply a clue to the acupuncturist as to how to treat the patient in order to restore him to health, but nothing more.

Here, then, is the basic difference between orthodox drug

therapy and acupuncture. A patient who is prescribed drugs for his condition may be lucky first time – many are – and rapidly obtain relief, but some may have to try a succession of possible treatments before they get any worthwhile improvement in their condition. However, a patient being treated by an expert acupuncturist who can make a correct holistic diagnosis will be given treatment that is tailored for him, from the very beginning. Another major difference is that, in many cases of chronic illness, such as arthritis, chronic bronchitis or psoriasis, the patient who is treated by orthodox means may have to remain on medication for life, since the drugs, although possibly controlling the symptoms admirably, may have no effect on the underlying condition. Acupuncture and other holistic therapies, which treat the body in such a way as to raise it to a level of energy at which it can heal itself, may, with expert treatment, reverse chronic diseases to a certain extent. Following a successful course of treatment it may be months or even years before the patient needs to see his practitioner again.

It must be said, of course, that not every patient will respond to acupuncture, even in expert hands. Here again, the patient is an individual and, in the same way that there is no one drug that suits every patient, there is no one therapy that suits everyone. Indeed, for those patients who do respond well to orthodox therapy, there would seem to be no advantage in looking elsewhere. But for those patients who are seeking an alternative therapy the business of finding the best treatment for them personally may, in fact, have a hit-and-miss element about it.

Chi

The Chinese see the whole functioning of the body and mind as being dependent on the normal flow of body energies, or life force, which they call Chi. In recent years, a new way of interpreting Chinese words into Roman characters has been used and, nowadays, Chi is sometimes spelled Qi or Ki. However, since, in English, the word is usually pronounced 'chee', I prefer to retain the older spelling.

Chi, then, is the life force, but not just the life force of the individual person or animal, and my Chi is not distinct from your Chi. Chi is a universal energy which surrounds and pervades everything, both animate and inanimate. Like radio waves or ultraviolet light, we cannot see Chi, nor can we feel it. Like these other two energies, we can only recognize it in terms of what it causes to happen. Radio waves, when picked up by a receiver tuned into the right frequency, will transmit sound. But a radio through which radio waves do not pass cannot, of itself, produce any sounds. In the same way, Chi is apparent to us as the life force of a body, and a body which no longer has Chi circulating through it is dead. But, in the same way that radio waves do not depend on the existence of radio sets for their existence and therefore do not disappear when a set is broken, so the Chi that permeates a body does not just disappear at its death. Chi is in a constant state of flux; there is constant interchange between the Chi of the body and Chi of the environment or external Chi. And, in the same way that food can be good or bad, nourishing or poisonous, external Chi can also be good or harmful.

Like air and food, Chi is taken in from the outside, in conjunction with these in the processes of breathing and eating. This external Chi is transformed within the body and is used to replenish one's own internal Chi. Waste Chi is eliminated in the same way as the end products of respiration and digestion. Within the body, Chi performs several specific functions, one of which is to form protective Chi. If this protective Chi is strong, it acts as a defence against any harmful external Chi with which one may come into contact. However, if one's protective Chi is weak, then one's resistance is lowered and one can be attacked by harmful external Chi. If this happens, the body becomes ill. This is a concept which is also understood, although in different terms, in Western medicine. Most people are aware that if they are 'run down' or overtired, or if their diet is poor, they are more likely to suffer from infections. What a nutritionist would call vitamin-rich food might be referred to by a Chinese physician as food rich in Chi. This is an interesting concept which can, to a certain extent, be demonstrated physically by Kirlian electrography, a method whereby an image is obtained on photographic paper of the energy (or 'corona discharge') emanating from a person or an object. It is commonly used as an adjunct to complementary therapies, when pictures taken of patients' hands and feet can aid in their diagnosis by pointing out abnormalities in the body's energy field. Pictures can also be obtained of inanimate objects and it has been found that foods that have high nutritional values, such as green vegetables and wholemeal bread, have a much better corona discharge than 'junk' foods which contain few vitamins or minerals. Whether what the pictures show as a discharge is what the Chinese know as Chi has not been proved as yet, but there is no doubt that when one eats nutritionally wholesome food, one is also ingesting some form of energy as well.

Thus the patient on a poor diet may be laying himself open to attack by lowering his defences. Stress, too, can break down our resistance to illness, and Chinese medical theory recognizes that not all disease comes from outside as an attack by harmful Chi, but may also be due to problems arising within – often arising from emotional problems.

Whether or not we get ill depends not just on the germs, carcinogens and other outside influences available to attack us but also, and more importantly, on our own inner resistance – or protective Chi. This idea is not alien to the thinking of Western physicians, although, of course, they express it in different terms. In his book *Cancer and Its Nutritional Therapies*, Dr Richard A. Passwater writes that 'fanatical avoidance of every possible carcinogen is not possible. They are everywhere ... The best hope remains in always retaining a strong immune response.'

Whether one thinks in terms of Chi or of immune response, once we have become ill, our inner resistance is also of vital importance in determining how easily and quickly we get better. By raising the patient's level of health, one can reinforce his intrinsic resistance to disease and thus he can be helped to heal himself.

Some people, of course, just never seem to get ill whereas others are always laid low by every bug that's going. This is beautifully illustrated by a scene in one of my favourite films, *The Apartment*, starring Jack Lemmon and Shirley MacLaine. Fairly early on in the film, Jack Lemmon catches a streaming cold after he has been shut out of his apartment for the best part of the night in the pouring rain. Going into work in the morning (he is a clerk in a huge New York insurance company), he steps into the lift to go up to his floor and tells the lift-girl (Shirley MacLaine) not to stand too close for fear of catching his germs.

'I never get colds,' says she, casually. Jack Lemmon is impressed by this. He tells her that he has been looking at the statistics on colds and asks, 'Did you know that the average New Yorker between twenty and fifty has two and a half colds a year?'

'That makes me feel just terrible,' says Shirley MacLaine.

'Why?' asks Lemmon.

'Well, to make the figures come out even, if I have no colds a year, some poor slob must have five colds a year.'

'Yes,' agrees Lemmon, 'it's me.'

In Chinese terms, people like the character played by Jack Lemmon are out of balance, whereas Shirley MacLaine's lift-girl and others like her are in balance. If Shirley MacLaine had stayed out all night in the rain she probably wouldn't have caught a cold, or, at most, she would have developed just a temporary sniffle. People like this have strong protective Chi. They are taking in plenty of good Chi to replenish their internal Chi. And Chi is circulating round their bodies normally, not encountering any blockages, and with perfect balance between its opposing positive and negative aspects, yin and yang.

Yin and Yang

Like Chi, yin and yang pervade everything. However, unlike Chi, they are not energies in themselves but are aspects of everything, each being unable to exist without the other. One can think of them in the same terms as right and left: neither can be described without reference to the other and yet, as a pair, they are totally understandable and useful concepts. Yin and yang each have their own qualities and, because these qualities are the opposite of each other, yin and yang must be in perfect balance within the body in order to maintain perfect health. An imbalance will cause malfunction in the same way that an object that is much larger and heavier on the right than on the left may well topple over.

Yin pertains to coldness, slowness, dimness, quietness and solidity and is associated with female characteristics and with the night. Yang, on the other hand, is hot, fast, bright, excited and insubstantial and is associated with the male characteristics and with daytime. Anything that is interior, low down or moving in a downward direction is yin. Anything that is exterior, high up or moving upwards is yang.

However, because there is balance in everything, nothing is exclusively yin or exclusively yang, although it may be predominantly so. There is something of each aspect in everybody and everything. Although a man is predominantly yang in his make-up, he has some balancing yin; similarly, a woman has a predominance of yin, but she still has a yang component.

Western medicine, too, recognizes that women have a male component and men a female component. It is known, of course, that the sex of a foetus is determined at conception, with the fusion of an egg with a sperm carrying an X chromosome resulting in a girl, while fusion with a Y-carrying sperm produces a boy. However, in the early stages, all embryos develop in the same way, regardless of which sex they will ultimately be. The sexual organs develop from the same cells, whether the baby is a boy or a girl, and it is at a fairly late stage of intra-uterine development that physical differentiation takes place. At birth, all babies are roughly the same shape and, with their nappies on, it is often hard to tell boys from girls. The typical body shape and hair distribution of male and female develop in response to the hormones that they secrete and, because males can secrete some female hormones and females can secrete some male hormones, it is possible for women to become hairy or for men to develop breast tissue. This can sometimes be seen as a result of quite normal development at puberty, while the hormones are 'sorting themselves out'.

One could say that the hairy girl had a temporary excess of yang, while the boy whose breasts began to swell would have excessive yin. But the terms yin and yang encompass far more than just sexual characteristics. As components of all animate and inanimate objects, they are in a constant state of flux and, according to how one looks at something, so its 'yin-ness' and 'yang-ness' change. For example, when one looks at the body as a whole, the outside surface (being exterior) is yang and the inner organs (known as the zang-fu organs) are yin. But if one looks only at the trunk, the back is primarily yang and the chest and abdomen (being the front, or the 'inside' when one bends over) are yin. But, there again, if one looks at the chest and abdomen, the chest can be said to be yang, being upper, and the abdomen, being lower, is yin. Thus it can be seen that yin and yang are not concrete characteristics of an object but are more relevant to that object's relationships to whatever is surrounding it. Here again, the comparison with the concepts of left and right is useful. If you describe your body, you will describe one arm as the left arm and the other as the right arm. However, you could also describe the inside border of your right arm as its left border, or the inside border of your left arm as its right border. So that which is right has an aspect of leftness and vice versa. Similarly, because we always look at our own bodies from a looking forward position, our right and left arms remain constant. But if we look at our environment, right and left are variable – Myrtle Crescent may be the first on the left past the church or the last on the right before the church, depending on where we are standing when we give the directions.

In all things that are opposite aspects of each other, there has to be balance, since, by definition, it is the two together that make the whole. Thus one could not have right without left, nor could one recognize light without knowledge of darkness. And the balance which is essential within the body must also be maintained between the body and its environment.

In Western medical terms, a fairly simple example of this can be given. Sixty per cent of our bodies are made up of water, and this water is distributed throughout the body. A certain amount of it is inside the body cells, some makes up the interstitial fluids which flow round and between the cells, keeping them moist, and the rest is in the body fluids – the blood, lymph, saliva, digestive juices and other secretions. It is very important that the amount of water in each section remains constant in relation to the others. The body would not be able to function if, when water was drunk, it flowed into a section in a haphazard way. For example, if excess water entered the blood, the increased blood volume could cause high blood pressure. Similarly, if too much water entered the tissue cells, these would swell causing oedema (swelling of the tissues). So the body has highly complex mechanisms by which the amount of water taken in is apportioned in the correct amounts to the various places where it is needed, and so it remains balanced.

Anything that has to keep a balance cannot be static or rigid, because it must always be ready to adapt to changes occurring around it. The balance of yin and yang must always be fluid. It follows, therefore, that any condition which restricts this fluidity will affect the body's ability to maintain its own natural health. In Chinese terms, many medical problems are associated with an imbalance of yin and yang. One may be in excess, or one may be deficient. If yin becomes excessive it will overwhelm the yang which is trying to balance it. This will result in a disease which has the characteristics of yin: coldness, slowness and lack of activity. But the same type of disease can result if the excess of yin is only relative – in other words, if it is due to a deficiency of yang. In the same way, an excess of yang will overwhelm normal yin producing a disease with yang characteristics – heat, excitement and overactivity, which can also be symptoms of a lack of yin.

To someone with a Western medical training, who was not looking at the patient in terms of yin and yang, a patient with a deficiency of yang could appear to have an identical illness to a patient suffering from an excess of yin. After doing various tests, the physician might diagnose a case of myxoedema, or thyroid deficiency, in which these physical signs are commonly found, and treat the patient with a thyroid supplement. However, if a patient with myxoedema were to be seen by an acupuncturist, he could be diagnosed as having either an excess of yin or a deficiency of yang. And the acupuncturist would treat the patient with excessive yin differently from one with deficient yang, since he would try to bring back to normal the aspect which was malfunctioning.

The Chinese term for excess, or fullness, is shi, and that for deficiency, or emptiness, is xu. Disease states in which the fundamental problém is an excess (whatever the excess may be of) are known as shi syndromes while those in which there is a deficiency of any sort are known as xu syndromes. A shi syndrome may be seen as one in which, although its natural resistance is intact, the body has been invaded and overwhelmed by an outside agent, while a xu syndrome is one in which the body's own defences have been lowered to such an extent that it has no resistance. It is clear, therefore, why treatment of the two types of syndrome must differ from each other: in a xu syndrome it is necessary to reinforce the body's defences against invasion – for example, if yin is deficient then it must be stimulated; in a shi syndrome, however, the treatment is to reduce the excessive factor.

A parallel can be found in Western medical terms. The white blood cells are the body's protection against infection. The production of these cells is dependent on a number of factors, not least on one's dietary intake of certain essential factors, such as vitamins C and E, zinc and magnesium. If one gets an infection, it may be because the white blood cells are deficient or because the bacteria are too strong for the body's defences. In the latter case (a 'shi' syndrome) antibiotics would be needed to fight the bacteria, but in the former (a 'xu' syndrome) it might only be necessary to supplement the patient's diet so that his natural defences were reinforced (such as many people do when they take large doses of vitamin C to treat a cold).

A disruption in the balance between yin and yang, whether it is due to an excess or a deficiency, produces an abnormality in the flow of Chi in the affected area. When the balance of yin and yang is restored to normal, the flow of Chi will also return to normal.

Chi itself can be divided into categories according to the function that it is performing. Having previously said that Chi is all-pervading and is in a constant state of flux, this may sound contradictory. However, a parallel with blood may make this clearer. The composition of one person's blood remains the same in terms of the number of red blood cells, white cells and platelets in it, and in terms of the amount of iron in the red cells, no matter where in the body that blood is. However, other things about it will vary according to what its function is at the time. Arterial blood, which has just left the lungs, is carrying oxygen to the body tissues and will be bright red, while venous blood, which is returning to the lungs and is carrying carbon dioxide to be exhaled, is dark red. Portal venous blood will contain breakdown products of protein, fat and carbohydrate which it carries from the intestines to the liver, while blood entering the kidneys will contain waste products from the body cells. But, fundamentally, it is all the same blood and that which is venous one minute can be arterial the next simply by passing through the lungs. Similarly, Chi can be divided into categories. Because it pervades everything, it is seen as being taken in with food and with the air one breathes. Inhaled air contains clean Chi, exhaled air contains waste Chi. These, together with the nutrients obtained from food, are known as material Chi. Nourishing Chi is derived from the digestion of food by the stomach and spleen and circulates through the meridians which, like the arteries and veins which carry the blood, carry Chi around the body. It is these meridians that form the basis for acupuncture therapy. Protecting Chi, which we have mentioned as being the body's natural defence against invasion, is also formed from food and circulates in the superficial tissues of the body and in the skin. Nourishing Chi is primarily yin, whereas protecting Chi is primarily yang – again, two aspects of the same thing.

Each organ of the body has its own Chi, which is known as functional Chi, and it is this that maintains the normal function of that organ. However, all these different forms of Chi are interrelated and interdependent, in exactly the same way that venous blood becomes arterial blood after it has been through the lungs, and arterial blood becomes venous blood after it has delivered its oxygen to the tissues. The purpose of protective Chi is to help to defend the body from attack by harmful Chi, which can invade the body and cause illness. By stimulating and strengthening the level of protective Chi, acupuncture can be used as a preventive treatment.

The Meridians

Acupuncture treatment uses as its medium the meridians through which Chi flows. The meridians may be thought of as being similar to the blood vessels, with an identical supply to the right and left sides of the body. In the same way that there is a right carotid artery and a left carotid artery, a right renal artery and a left renal artery, a right femoral vein and a left femoral vein, and so on, so there are right and left Lung meridians, right and left Kidney meridians, and so on. There is, however, a difference. If, for example, there is a malfunction of a vein on the left, in orthodox medicine, it is the left vein that will be treated, whereas in acupuncture, treatment of either the left or right meridian of the pair will affect the other. Some authorities state that to treat only the opposite meridian to the one affected will produce an effect in 30 per cent of cases, to treat only the affected meridian will produce an effect in 60 per cent, and treatment of both together will produce an effect in 90 per cent. Other practitioners, more cynical perhaps, say that the reason for this is that if one is inaccurate in locating the acupuncture points, then treatment of both sides gives an increased chance of actually hitting the right spot! Be this as it may, some practitioners will always treat the patient symmetrically. The fact that treatment of the opposite meridian will affect the disturbed meridian is very valuable when one is treating a patient in whom pain makes it impossible to treat the affected side – for example, someone suffering from shingles, in whom the needles would commonly be put on the opposite side of the body to the rash.

There are twelve pairs of meridians in which each half of the pair behaves exactly like its partner, unless one of them is diseased. It is easier, however, to speak of 'the Lung meridian' than of 'the two Lung meridians, left and right'. This, therefore, is the terminology that is commonly used and that will be used in the rest of this book.

In addition to the twelve major meridians, there are two unpaired meridians, known as Du and Ren, which run down the midline of the body, back and front. There are also six other 'extra' meridians which are made up of points from the major meridians and form links between them. And the meridians are joined to each other by collaterals which can be used to carry excess Chi from one meridian which has too much to another which is deficient.

Each of the twelve major meridians is associated with an organ of the body – thus we have the Lung meridian, the Liver meridian, the Heart meridian and so on. Each meridian receives Chi from another meridian and passes it on to a third, so that Chi circulates around the meridians in the same way that blood circulates through the blood vessels. However, where the circulation of the blood is concerned, the amount of blood in a vessel at any one time varies. For example, after a meal, there will be an increased amount of blood in the vessels supplying the stomach and intestines. Or, when the weather is hot, there will be an increased supply to the skin so that heat can be lost from the body (causing the flushed face characteristic of someone who is overheated). The flow of Chi through the meridians, however, is controlled by a strict 'biological clock'.

Chi is said to surge in individual meridians at particular times. Each of the twelve major meridians is coupled with one of the others and, while Chi is surging in one of the couple, it will be at its lowest ebb in the other. Thus, Chi is said to be at its maximum in the Liver meridian between 1.00 and 3.00 in the morning, while its opposite number, the Small Intestine meridian, is at its lowest during this period. Between 1.00 and 3.00 in the afternoon, however, the position is reversed, with the Small Intestine meridian having its maximum flow of Chi and the Liver meridian its lowest.

It has been suggested that jet lag may be due to the meridians not having yet adapted to the new time zone in which they have arrived – going from London to New York will find the Liver meridian having its maximum flow at around 8.00 in the evening, instead of in the early hours of the morning, which is what it is used to. The meridians adapt fairly rapidly in a healthy person but, until they do so, he may feel somewhat out of sorts.

The theory of the circulation of Chi is of use to the acupuncturist both in the diagnosis and in the treatment of his patient. For example, a patient suffering from ulcerative colitis may often be woken by abdominal pain and a desire to have his bowels open at around 5.00 or 6.00 in the morning. To the acupuncturist, the symptoms, plus the timing, suggest a disruption of the Large Intestine meridian, which has its maximum flow of Chi between 5.00 and 7.00 a.m. It is sometimes helpful, if possible, to treat a meridian during its period of maximum flow and a patient may therefore be asked to make an appointment for a particular time of day. Obviously, this is more likely to be done with the meridians that have their surges of flow during the day rather than with those that peak at night, since acupuncturists, like doctors, are unlikely to treat anything other than emergencies at night.

Each meridian is predominantly either yin or yang (although, of course, each will have aspects of both). In the coupling of meridians, each yin meridian is associated with a yang meridian so that, when Chi is at its maximum in a yin meridian, it is at its lowest in a yang one and vice versa. The circulation of Chi around the meridians entails it passing through two yin meridians, followed by two yang meridians, then two yin meridians, and so on. Each yin meridian is associated with a so-called solid (or zang) organ, while yang meridians are associated with hollow (or fu) organs. This relates back to the association of yin with solidity and yang with lack of substance.

When looked at anatomically, not all the 'solid' organs are truly solid so it might be more appropriate to refer to them by the Chinese terms, zang and fu. The zang organs are the heart, the liver, the spleen, the lung, the kidney and the pericardium (the fibrous sac that surrounds the heart and assists its contraction and which in some Western books on acupuncture is referred to as the heart constrictor). The fu organs are the small intestine, the large intestine, the stomach, the gall bladder, the urinary bladder and the sanjiao or triple warmer. The latter is a Chinese concept and is not an organ in its own right in Western terms. The word sanjiao may be translated as 'three warmers'. The term refers to the chest (or upper jiao), the upper abdomen (the middle jiao) and the lower abdomen (the lower jiao),

which are related to each other by their function of warming the organs contained within them.

The routes taken by the meridians are also related to
their yin or yang qualities. For example, yin meridians of
the arm run down its inner aspect, yang meridians down
the outside.

Each meridian is related internally with the organ from
which it gets its name, for example, the Lung meridian
extends into the lungs, the Liver meridian into the liver and
the Large Intestine meridian into the large bowel. The
organs themselves can be affected by treatment of the corresponding meridian and disorders of a particular meridian
may manifest as symptoms associated with its organ. In
other words, the organ and its meridian are intimately
related. The meridians that are shown in the diagrams tell
only half the story. They illustrate the part of the meridian
that is used in treatment – in other words, that part which
runs near the surface of the body and along which lie the
acupuncture points. However, these 'surface' meridians
extend into internal meridians which are the links between
the acupuncture points (those sites into which needles are
inserted during treatment) and the internal organs.

The Lung meridian is a yin meridian and runs, super-
ficially, from just below the collar bone, down the inside of
the arm and into the thumb, where it ends just next to the
nail. This is shown in Figure 1. When the meridians are
listed, the Lung meridian is usually put first since it is seen
as being the starting point in the cycle of Chi. It has its
surge of energy between 3.00 and 5.00 a.m., at which time
its coupled meridian, that of the Urinary Bladder, is at its
lowest. There are eleven acupuncture points lying along the
course of the meridian and these are referred to either by
their Chinese names or else as Lung 1, Lung 2, and so on,
often abbreviated to Lu 1, Lu 2.

Interruption of the flow of Chi in the Lung meridian, and

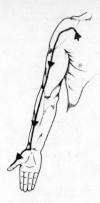

Figure 1

thus disruption of its function, may be associated with various chest symptoms, such as cough, asthma or tightness in the chest (associated with the internal course of the meridian and its link with the lungs) or with symptoms in the arm, along the course of the superficial part of the meridian. When it affects a single meridian, either wholly or predominantly, an excess of Chi may produce certain diagnostic symptoms, as may a deficiency. These are related to the function and course of the meridian itself. (More will be said about excess and deficiency syndromes in the next chapter.) When the Lung meridian is concerned, an excess may produce symptoms of a heavy feeling in the chest, shortness of breath, a severe cough with copious sputum, a dry and sore throat, a nasal discharge, redness of the bridge of the nose and pain in the shoulder and arm. A deficiency may result in sneezing, a dry cough, dry skin, faintness, weight loss, shallow breathing, sensitivity to cold and redness of the chin.

Figure 2 shows the Large Intestine meridian, which is the first of the two yang meridians that come immediately after the Lung meridian in the daily cycle of Chi. It surges

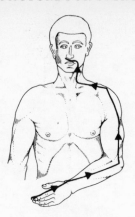

Figure 2

between 5.00 and 7.00 a.m., when the Kidney meridian, with which it is coupled, is at its lowest. Because the Large Intestine meridian receives Chi directly from the Lung meridian, it begins very close to the end of the latter, its first point being next to the nail of the index finger. Being a yang meridian, in its course up the arm it runs up the outside aspect. Since it terminates so close to the nose, disruption of this meridian may be associated with nosebleeds. In addition, because it passes across the lower part of the face, it may be associated with toothache. Sore throat and pain in the shoulder or arm are associated with the position of the rest of its superficial course. And because of its internal links with the large intestine itself, abdominal pain and diarrhoea may also be involved with disruption of this meridian. An excess in the meridian is likely to cause pain along its course, stiffness of the shoulder, dizziness, abdominal distension and constipation, while a deficiency may result in diarrhoea, shivering and a dry mouth. The Large Intestine meridian has twenty points along its superficial course, which are listed as L I 1, L I 2, and so on. In some books, the meridian is called the Colon meridian

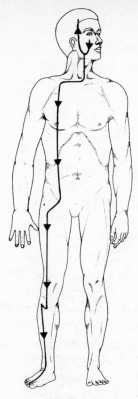

Figure 3

(colon being another name for the greater part of the large intestine) and in this case the abbreviation is Co 1, Co 2 and so on.

From the Large Intestine meridian, Chi runs down the yang Stomach meridian, which is shown in Figure 3. Here again, the fact that it is a yang meridian is reflected in its course which, when it runs down the leg, does so along the outer aspect. The Stomach meridian has its surge of Chi between 7.00 and 9.00 a.m., when the Pericardium meridian is at its lowest. Disruption of the flow of Chi in the Stomach meridian may produce symptoms associated with any part of its superficial course, such as nosebleeds, sore throat or chest pain. Symptoms related to the stomach itself, such as indigestion or upper abdominal pain, may also occur. An excess in the meridian may cause an increase in appetite, constipation, thirst, bad breath, swelling and pain in the mouth, cramps in the legs and fever. A deficiency may produce distension of the abdomen, diarrhoea, vomiting and loss of appetite, and weakness in the legs. Forty-five points lie along the Stomach meridian, abbreviated as St 1 to St 45.

The yin Spleen meridian continues the course of Chi, travelling from the big toe up the leg (along the inside, being a yin meridian) and over the abdomen to end a little way below the armpit. Its course is shown in Figure 4. Interference with its function may cause vomiting, upper abdominal pain, jaundice or diarrhoea, all of which are related to its internal course and its path across the abdomen, or it may produce symptoms lower down in its course, such as painful or swollen knees. An excess affecting this meridian is likely to cause congestion in the chest with a productive cough, constipation, fatigue and an irregular appetite. A deficiency may cause diarrhoea and vomiting, flatulence, water retention, sleepiness, heaviness of the legs and a poor memory. The surge of Chi in this meridian comes between 9.00 and 11.00 a.m., the Sanjiao meridian having the lowest flow at this time. Like the Large Intestine meridian, the Spleen meridian has twenty points, abbreviated as Sp 1 to Sp 20.

From the end of the Spleen meridian, Chi is taken up by the yin Heart meridian which runs from the armpit, down the inside of the arm and into the little finger, as shown in Figure 5. Figure 6 shows how, from the little finger, it flows out again via the yang Small Intestine meridian, up the outer (yang) aspect of the arm, finally finishing just in front

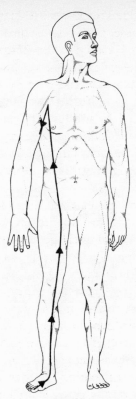

Figure 4

of the ear. The Heart meridian is one of the two shortest
meridians, with only nine points along its course, abbreviated to H 1, H 2 and so on. Disruption of this meridian
can cause symptoms which tie in well with the Western
concept of heart disease, such as chest pain, palpitations
and pain in the arms, but, because the heart in Chinese
medicine is said to be the seat of the mind, it can also produce symptoms such as insomnia. An excess may be associated with a feeling of heaviness in the chest and a fever,
while a deficiency may cause cold sweats, restlessness,

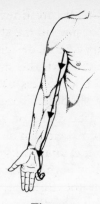

Figure 5

palpitations and a poor memory. The Chi flowing through the Heart meridian, which is coupled with the Gall Bladder meridian, surges between 11.00 a.m. and 1.00 p.m.

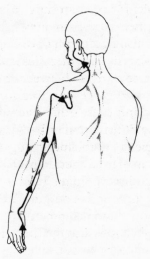

Figure 6

Disruption of the Small Intestine meridian may produce deafness, sore throat or pain in the shoulder and arm, all of which are related to its course, or abdominal pain, which is related to its inner links with the small bowel. Cold sores may be associated with an excess in this meridian, as may pain in the neck and shoulder. Ringing in the ears and a tender abdomen may be signs of a deficiency. Nineteen points lie along its course, shown as SI 1 to SI 19. Chi in the Small Intestine meridian surges between 1.00 and 3.00 p.m., when the flow in the Liver meridian is lowest.

Following on from the Small Intestine meridian, the yang Urinary Bladder meridian takes Chi from the area between the eye and the nose, up across the head and down through the neck and along the side of the spine to the leg, where it travels down the back of the leg and into the foot to finish in the little toe. Its route is shown in Figure 7. As can be seen, the Urinary Bladder meridian also has an extra branch which runs parallel to the first channel down the length of the spine.

Urinary problems are, naturally, associated with malfunction of this meridian. Pain anywhere along the length of the spine may also be a result of disruption of the flow of Chi in the Urinary Bladder meridian. Because the channel starts its external course just between the nose and the eye, injury to it may also be responsible for nasal congestion, nosebleeds, watering eyes, other eye problems and headaches. Frequency of urination or bed-wetting may occur as a result of a deficiency in the meridian. It was mentioned in connection with its paired meridian, that of the Lung, that the Urinary Bladder meridian was at its lowest ebb of energy between 3.00 and 5.00 a.m. This, of course, is a period of the night that is commonly associated with bed-wetting in children and is also the time at which many older people find it necessary to get up in order to pass water. The surge of energy in the Urinary Bladder meridian

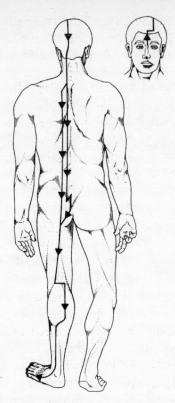

Figure 7

comes at the opposite end of the day, between 3.00 and 5.00 in the afternoon. This is the longest of the meridians, mainly due to its parallel tracks down the vertebral column. There are sixty-seven points, which are commonly abbreviated to UB1, UB2, and so on. However, like the Large Intestine (or Colon) meridian, the Urinary Bladder meridian has an alternative name and some books refer to it simply as the Bladder meridian. The numbering of points along the meridian is not consistent in all books, either. Some authorities (usually Chinese) number the points from the eye down to the base of the spine as UB 1 to UB 35, then from below the buttock to the knee as UB 36 to UB 40, the parallel course in the back as UB 41 to UB 54 and, finally, from below the knee to the end of the meridian as UB 55 to UB 64. The other system of numbering, which seems to be favoured in America, is to number from the eye to the base of the spine in the same way, as UB 1 to UB 35, then the parallel course in the back as UB 36 to UB 49 and, carrying straight on down, through the buttock, to the knee and foot with UB 50 to 67.

The next meridian in the cycle, which is shown in Figure 8, is the yin Kidney meridian. It begins, as may be guessed, near the termination of the Urinary Bladder meridian, in the foot. It starts on the sole of the foot and runs up the leg (along the inside, being a yin channel) and then up the abdomen, near the midline, to finish just below the inner aspect of the collar bone. It has its surge of energy between 5.00 and 7.00 p.m. and the twenty-seven points that lie along its course are abbreviated to K 1 to K 27.

Urinary problems are, of course, associated with abnormalities of the Kidney meridian, as well as of the Urinary Bladder meridian. However, the former also regulates the sexual function and so disruption of its flow of Chi may cause menstrual problems in women and impotence in men. Its course across the chest means that asthma, coughing of blood and sore throat may all be associated with problems in the Kidney meridian, and its course down the legs may produce local pain as a symptom of malfunction. An excess in the meridian may cause the patient to become hyperactive, while a deficiency can produce a loss of sex drive and a general timidity; both may be associated with ringing in the ears (more will be said about the kidney's association with the ears later on).

Following on from the Kidney meridian is the yin Pericardium meridian which is illustrated in Figure 9. The

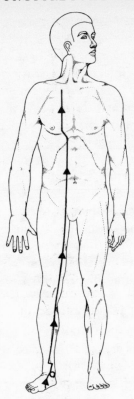

Figure 8

yang Sanjiao meridian, shown in Figure 10, then carries
Chi from the ring finger, up the arm (the outer aspect, since
it is a yang meridian), into the shoulder, up the side of the
neck, and around the ear to finish next to the outside end of
the eyebrow. The Pericardium meridian, like the Heart
meridian, with which it is closely associated, has only nine
points, listed as P1 to P9 or, in some books, as HC1 to
HC9, where HC stands for Heart Constrictor. The
Sanjiao meridian is another which has two names, with its
twenty-three points listed either as SJ1 to SJ23, or as

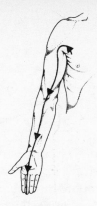

Figure 9

TH 1 to TH 23, TH being the abbreviation for 'Triple Heater'. Chi surges through the Pericardium meridian between 7.00 and 9.00 p.m. and through the Sanjiao meridian between 9.00 and 11.00 p.m.

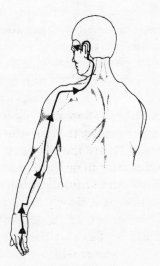

Figure 10

It can be seen from Figure 9 that the Pericardium meridian runs more or less parallel with the Heart meridian. It is associated with heart problems, since the heart itself is contained within the pericardium. These problems include chest pain, palpitations and shortness of breath. Malfunction of the Pericardium meridian can also produce anxiety and mental disturbance (associated with the heart being the seat of the mind). Headache, abdominal pains and fever may be associated with an excess affecting the Pericardium meridian, while a deficiency may cause palpitations, shortness of breath, indigestion and diarrhoea; both may result in restless sleep. Disruption of the Sanjiao meridian can cause problems associated with any of the three cavities. For example, abdominal pain or distension may relate to the middle cavity or jiao, and pain on passing urine to the lower jiao. However, the superficial route of the meridian is not across the area that it regulates and symptoms may simply be related to its course – for example, ringing in the ears, sore throat or pain in the shoulders or arms. Pain in the shoulders and arms may relate to an excess in the meridian, as may a sore throat, hearing difficulties, constipation and retention of urine. A deficiency can be associated with nervousness and restlessness, diarrhoea, incontinence or water retention.

The yang Gall Bladder meridian, whose energy surges between 11.00 p.m. and 1.00 a.m., follows on from the Sanjiao meridian. Its long and somewhat convoluted route is shown in Figure 11. Here again, it will be noted that, being a yang meridian, it runs down the outside of the leg. Disruption of the flow of Chi may cause symptoms related to any part of its superficial course, such as headache, blurring of vision, chest or upper abdominal pain and pain in the legs. An excess in the meridian may produce an increased appetite, abdominal pain or jaundice, while a deficiency may be responsible for dizziness, anxiety and

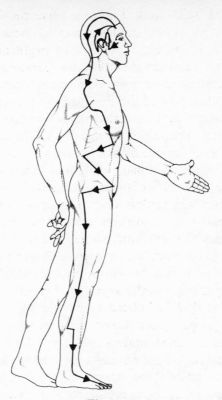

Figure 11

insomnia. Forty-four points lie along its course and are abbreviated to GB 1, GB 2, and so on.

The Liver meridian is a yin meridian and runs, as can be seen in Figure 12, from the big toe, up the inside of the leg to the trunk where it ends just below the nipple. This meridian is at its highest point of energy between 1.00 and 3.00 in the morning. Disruption of the function of the Liver meridian may be associated with pain anywhere along its superficial course, but particularly with pain in the lower

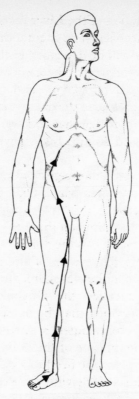

Figure 12

abdomen and pain on passing water. Its course passes through the groin and therefore hernias may be associated with its malfunction. So, too, may a feeling of tightness in the lower part of the chest, and hiccups (which are due to spasmodic contractions of the diaphragm – a large sheet of muscle that is attached to the lower border of the ribs and that separates the abdomen from the chest). The liver is said to have specific functions, which are not the same as those accorded it in Western medicine, and these may be disrupted by malfunction of the Liver meridian, producing symptoms such as headache and mental disturbance. (The functions of the liver will be described in the next chapter.) An excess in the meridian may be associated with an unstable temperament, hyperactivity and abdominal pain, while a deficiency may cause dizziness, poor eyesight and dry skin. The Liver meridian has fourteen points, usually abbreviated to Liv 1 to Liv 14, but shown as Li in some books.

From the Liver meridian, the circulation of Chi is completed by the Lung meridian which takes it up again from under the collar bone.

The total number of points on these twelve meridians is 309 although, of course, this is the number of points on just one side of the body. Since each of the meridians is bilateral, there are 618 points available for use. The Du meridian (sometimes called the Governing Vessel and abbreviated to GV), which may be associated with back pain and headache, contributes a further twenty-eight points. It runs up the midline of the body from a point at the base of the spine, over the head to a point in the centre of the top lip. It forms a circle with the Ren meridian, also known as the Vessel of Conception and abbreviated to VC, or even CV. This meridian is associated with menstrual problems, vaginal discharge, retention of urine, and abdominal pain. The Ren meridian has twenty-four points along its course which runs from a point in the centre of the perineum (the area in front of the anus and between the legs), up the midline of the abdomen and chest, to finish just below the centre of the lower lip. The course of these two meridians is shown in Figures 13 and 14.

The 'extra' meridians are made up of points from the other main meridians and thus serve to link them. For example, the Yangwei meridian (a yang meridian, naturally) runs through points on the yang Urinary Bladder,

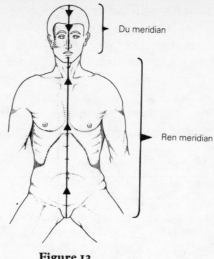

Figure 13

Gall Bladder, Small Intestine, Sanjiao, Stomach and Du meridians, while the Yingwei meridian (a yin meridian) joins points on the yin Kidney, Spleen, Liver and Ren meridians. The Du meridian is yang since it runs down the back, or outside, of the body, while the Ren meridian, running down the inside, is yin.

There are also twenty extra points which are not connected with any specific meridian. Since Chi must, by its nature, circulate through the entire body, an acupuncture point does not necessarily have to be on a meridian, in the same way that one does not have to cut through a vein or artery in order to bleed.

The total number of acupuncture points from the twelve meridians, the two midline meridians and the extra points is $309 + 28 + 24 + 20 = 381$. (Modern researchers have discovered a large number of 'extra' points, though 381 is still

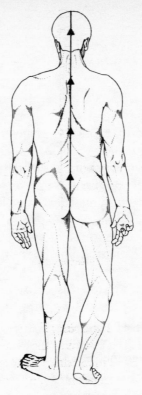

Figure 14

considered the basic figure.) It is interesting to recall that the *Nei Ching* refers to 365 points, demonstrating that very little has changed in the basic theory of acupuncture in 2000 years.

THE FIVE ELEMENTS

Although the meridians vary as to the number of acupuncture points that they incorporate, some being much longer than others, each of the twelve major meridians has five points that relate to the five elements. In classical Chinese philosophy the five elements are understood to be earth, wood, water, metal and fire and they are seen as being intimately associated with all things, including the human body. As well as having the five points that are associated with the elements, each of the meridians is itself associated with a particular element. Sometimes the reasoning behind the association is obvious, even to Western eyes. For example, the Heart meridian is a Fire meridian, since it is associated with the idea of heat, and the Urinary Bladder and Kidney meridians are, of course, Water meridians. Some of the other associations, however, are not quite so logical. The five elements are distributed among twelve meridians, four of which are associated with fire, while the other elements have two each.

These five elements are related to each other in various ways and their relationships are governed by the Law of the Five Elements. Because each meridian is associated with an individual element, the meridians are thus related to each other in exactly the same way as the elements to which they belong. Therefore, the meridians and the flow of Chi between them are also governed by the Law of the Five Elements (see Figure 15).

According to this law, each of the elements has an effect on the others, either directly or indirectly, and so disruption of one is likely to affect others. This is the basis of holistic practice: no one part of the body can be disrupted in any way, no matter how small, without its having an effect on other parts. The Law of the Five Elements, when applied to acupuncture practice, means that the meridian which is implicated by the symptoms that the patient is complaining of is not necessarily the meridian that needs treating. The underlying cause may be in another meridian whose disruption has caused abnormalities to occur in the symptom-producing meridian.

The rules that govern the effects of elements upon each other, and therefore of meridians upon each other, are known as the mother–child rule and the servant–master rule. It is said that, in the same way a mother gives birth to a child and nourishes it, so elements promote and nourish other elements. Wood is said to promote fire because it is combustible; a fire that is deprived of wood to burn will go out. Fire, in its turn, promotes earth by creating ashes. Even nowadays, certain forms of ash are used as fertilizers to nourish the earth. Earth promotes metal because metal is dug out of the earth and so is engendered by it. Metal promotes water – somewhat dubiously – by melting, and water promotes wood by nourishing the tree, for a tree that is deprived of water will die.

Thus, by analogy, when a meridian associated with Wood (that is, the Liver or the Gall Bladder meridian) is functioning normally, it will promote the normal flow of Chi and normal function in the Fire meridians (Heart, Pericardium, Small Intestine and Sanjiao). In turn, the normal function of the Fire meridians promotes normal function in the Earth meridians (Spleen and Stomach) which, in the same way, affect the Metal meridians (Lung and Large Intestine). These promote the function of the Water meridians (Urinary Bladder and Kidney) which complete the circle by affecting the Wood meridians.

It follows that disruption in the flow of Chi in one meridian can disrupt flow in the meridian that it normally promotes or nourishes. If the disruption is allowed to continue, untreated, it may go a step further, affecting the meridian that is nourished by the second meridian involved. Thus the condition can spread to involve the entire body and meridian system.

The servant–master rule produces a different cycle of events. It is said that, in the same way that a master gives orders to his servant and controls his actions, so elements affect others by maintaining control over them. It is this control by the master element, as much as the nourishment obtained from the mother element, that enables the element in question to function normally. Wood is said to control earth, since trees grow on it and over it. Earth in turn controls water by damming it and thus forcing it to flow in certain directions. Water controls fire, naturally enough, by extinguishing it, and fire controls metal by melting it. Metal controls wood by being made into tools that can cut it and fashion it into other things, and this completes the circle. Thus the Wood meridians (Liver and Gall Bladder) exert control over the Earth meridians (Spleen and Stomach). These two then control the Water meridians (Urinary Bladder and Kidney) which control the Fire meridians (Small Intestine, Sanjiao, Heart and Pericardium). The Fire meridians control the Metal meridians (Lung and Large Intestine) and the latter control the Wood meridians. A malfunction in a meridian may be produced by a malfunction in the master meridian which exerts either insufficient or excessive control over its servant. In the latter case, the function of the servant meridian may be reduced or, if the servant 'rebels' against the increased control, may be excessive.

Thus it can be seen that each meridian has four connections through the Law of the Five Elements. It is nourished by one meridian and controlled by another; it nourishes a third and controls a fourth. Therefore each element is con-

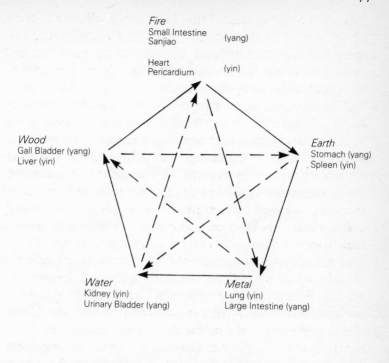

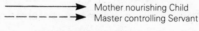

Mother nourishing Child
Master controlling Servant

Figure 15

nected with every other element, as shown in Figure 15, either as a mother, a child, a master or a servant. In this respect, the yin meridians primarily affect and are affected by the other yin meridians and the yang meridians primarily affect and are affected by the other yang meridians.

It may be helpful here to look at one meridian, for example the Heart meridian, and see how it can be affected by other meridians according to the mother–child and the servant–master rules. The Heart is a yin Fire meridian. It is nourished by its mother, the yin Wood meridian, and, in turn, nourishes its child, the yin Earth meridian. It is controlled by its master, the yin Water meridian, and itself controls its servant, the yin Metal meridian. This means that the Heart meridian is nourished by the Liver meridian, while giving nourishment to the Spleen meridian, and it is controlled by the Kidney meridian, while exerting control over the Lung meridian.

Thus a malfunction of the Heart meridian may be intimately related to a malfunction of the Liver, Spleen, Kidney or Lung meridians. If the disorder originated in one of the other meridians, then treatment of the Heart meridian alone will not resolve the problem. The whole system must be balanced before the body can become healthy again.

I have heard a Western medical practitioner say that he thought acupuncture must be an easy therapy to master, 'you just learn what each point does and then stick in your needles'. But what has just been said about the Law of the Five Elements should make it clear that this is not the case. Acupuncture is not about diseases but about energy flow. And therefore it is not a case of learning that 'this point cures headache and that one will stop vomiting'. Each point has a specific function, sure enough, but this function is to do with moving energies. And so, before one can use the points correctly, one has to have learned not only what each point does but how to make a diagnosis in terms of what has gone wrong with the energy flow. Admittedly, there are some points with specific action, such as the control of vomiting, but to use points only for their specific action without any knowledge of the theory of the flow of Chi is to use acupuncture at a fairly primitive level. The difference, perhaps, is that between a boy scout with a first-aid certificate and a consultant surgeon. The former may certainly have his uses in an emergency but one would not expect him to produce the same results as the surgeon and, indeed, if the boy scout tries to ape the surgeon's work, he may finish up doing more harm than good. If one is going to use acupuncture fully and correctly, in a truly holistic way, it takes at least three years to learn the basic theory. The skill of the acupuncturist lies in diagnosing where the imbalance of Chi is and, in order to do this, he has to know all the laws governing the behaviour of the meridians and of the Chi flowing in them. More will be said about diagnosis in the next chapter.

Let us return now to the Heart meridian which, as we have seen, is closely related through the Law of the Five Elements to the Liver, Spleen, Kidney and Lung meridians. According to this law, a deficiency of Chi in the Liver meridian, which is the mother meridian of the Heart meridian, could cause the latter to become undernourished so that it, too, would develop a deficiency of Chi. Similarly, an excess of Chi in the Liver meridian, could spill over and cause Chi in the Heart meridian to become excessive. A deficiency originating in the Heart meridian itself would deprive its child, the Spleen meridian. A condition in which a patient suffers from symptoms relating to one meridian (or element) which are the result of a deficiency in the mother of that meridian, is known as the 'screaming child syndrome' – and the child will go on screaming until it is nourished.

A deficiency in the Heart meridian could also track backwards in the cycle and produce a deficiency in the Liver meridian by 'sucking it dry'. An excess of Chi can also be transmitted either way, from mother to child or from child to mother. If there is found to be a deficiency, or an excess, in the Liver, Heart and Spleen meridians, this may well have originated from a primary disorder of the Heart meridian. In either case, treatment of the Heart meridian alone may resolve the problem.

The liver itself, as distinct from its meridian, is said, by

Chinese physicians, to store blood and to control the volume of the circulating blood. But the function of the liver is dependent on the normality of its related meridian. If there is a deficiency of Chi in the Liver meridian, not only Chi but blood may also be deficient and have an effect on its child, the Heart meridian, and therefore also on its related organ, the heart.

Western medicine also recognizes a link between the liver and the heart, although it is not expressed in the same terms as in Chinese medicine. The liver is the storehouse for various vitamins and minerals, including iron and vitamin B_{12}, which are essential for normal blood formation. A deficiency in the liver in Western terms (that is, a depletion of its nutritional stores) may have a serious effect on the blood, causing anaemia. This may then affect the action of the heart, which is put under stress in severe anaemia.

Another intimate relationship acknowledged by Western medicine links the spleen and the heart – the child and its mother, in Chinese terms. Red blood cells, which are the cells that actually carry oxygen in the blood, have a life span of about 120 days. Having reached this age, they are replaced by new cells and the old cells are broken down, the iron in them being reused in the bone marrow to form new cells. However, the breaking down of the old cells is done in the spleen. There are some forms of anaemia where excessive quantities of red blood cells are broken down, which are known as the haemolytic anaemias. Again, the heart may be affected, by being put under strain by the anaemia. Indeed, a sudden and overwhelming haemolytic crisis may precipitate heart failure. Although Chinese medicine does not describe the physiological function of the spleen in breaking down old red blood cells, it says that the spleen is the organ responsible for controlling the blood inside the blood vessels and preventing it from leaking out.

As we have seen, good health entails a normal balance

between the body energies and the Chi of all the meridians. If a meridian fails, it may lose its control over its servant meridian. Thus a failing Kidney meridian may lose control over its servant, the Heart meridian, or a failing Heart meridian, in the role of master, may lose control over the Lung meridian. The control exerted may be thought of as similar to that exerted physiologically by the pituitary gland over the other glands in the body. These glands work on what is known as a bio-feedback system. The pituitary gland secretes hormones which stimulate the other glands – adrenal glands, thyroid and ovaries or testes – to secrete their own hormones. When they do so, the increased level of hormones in the blood stream acts on the pituitary which then stops secreting the stimulating hormone and therefore regulates the secretions of the glands under its control. A patient with an overactive thyroid gland may have a problem either in the gland itself or in the pituitary gland which has, so to speak, lost control.

The servant–master relationship is therefore one in which overactivity or underactivity of a meridian or its related organ may be associated with a loss of control or an excess of control by the master meridian. The Kidney meridian controls the Heart meridian, and the Heart meridian controls the Lung meridian. These three organs, the kidney, heart and lung, are also recognized as being intimately related by Western physicians. The function of the kidneys is to maintain a balance of water and of minerals within the body. They also eliminate waste products, drugs and other toxins from the body, which they do by filtering the blood, removing waste, toxins, water and minerals, and then returning to the 'clean' blood exactly the right amount of water and minerals to keep the body in balance. The waste and rejected matter and the excess water are excreted as urine. If the kidneys fail to function normally, there is a build-up of toxins in the body, and retention of water and excessive minerals. The result is a rise in the blood pressure (seen, perhaps, in Chinese terms as a loss of control over the blood pressure). This affects the heart through its meridian, which, if one looks at it again in Chinese terms, is under the control of the Kidney meridian. A continued raised blood pressure may finally result in heart failure and this, in turn, causes fluid to accumulate in the lungs. In the West this would be called pulmonary oedema but, looked at through an acupuncturist's eyes, might be a case of the heart failing to control the lungs. As we shall see in the next chapter, the lung is one of the organs said by the Chinese to be responsible for the normal distribution of water around the body.

These relationships have been expressed here in rather simplistic terms; in both Western and Chinese medicine, the picture is rather more complicated. However, what can be shown is that, in both systems, the functions of these organs are interrelated.

The meridians which relate to each other as mother–child and servant–master, are linked by specific points, the needling of which can open a channel between the two in order to allow Chi to flow from one to the other and thus return to an equilibrium. Various points are available on each meridian by which transfer of Chi can be effected and every meridian has a point relating to each of the elements, earth, water, fire, metal and wood. These points are all to be found on the distal parts of the limbs: that is, on the meridians that run through the arms, the points are around and below the elbow; on those that run through the legs, they are around and below the knee. It is these points that may be used to transfer Chi to and from the related meridian associated with each element. Other points also have specific functions in terms of the transfer of Chi and particular effects on the meridian in question, and these will be mentioned later.

Over the thousands of years that acupuncture has been used in China, two major systems of diagnosis and treatment have developed. One is based entirely on the Law of the Five Elements. The other, while using this law, also diagnoses according to the Eight Conditions, or Eight Syndromes, which will be described in the next chapter. Because there are two systems, this does not mean that one is wrong and one is right, nor even that one is superior to the other. In acupuncture, the diagnosis is more a means to an end than a concrete entity. It is a signpost, indicating to the practitioner which points he should use in order to restore balance to the patient's body energies. Both systems work to restore the balance and both are effective in this respect, so that the fact that they achieve their results by working from different angles is not important.

In this book, I am going to concentrate mainly on diagnosis and treatment according to the Eight Syndromes, since this is the system with which I am the most familiar. However, in Chapter Seven, where I quote some case histories, I have been fortunate enough to be allowed to relate the histories of some patients treated by a practitioner who uses the Five Elements system. Before going on to explain the Eight Syndromes, I shall give a brief outline of the diagnosis used in the Five Elements system, which will help clarify these case histories.

When a practitioner of the Five Elements system makes a diagnosis, he does so according to the element which is disturbed. A patient is seen as having a susceptibility to injury to a particular element which may stem from trauma in childhood, or even from when he was still in the womb. Further trauma later in life is, therefore, likely to affect the meridians related to that element. Once this has occurred, the disturbance may spread to other meridians according to the mother–child and servant–master connections.

The practitioner will treat his patient in order to restore

balance between the meridians, to remove excess Chi or to stimulate a deficiency of Chi. His diagnosis is based on a number of factors such as the patient's colour, his voice, his emotions and his bodily odour.

A patient with a disturbance of the Wood element is likely to have a greenish look to his skin, a rancid odour and a loud aggressive voice. He may be irritable, restless and unstable and may be subject to depression.

If the Fire element is affected, the patient will have a red face, a 'scorched' bodily odour and a normal or laughing quality of voice. He may have very labile emotions, being up one minute and down the next.

The Earth patient has a yellowish look, a 'fragrant' bodily odour and a singing quality to his voice. He may be obsessional in nature, tense and overanxious, and may have a craving for sympathy.

A patient whose Metal meridians are affected will have a white complexion, a 'rotten' smell and a weeping quality of voice. He is likely to relate his story in grief-laden tones and to regard his problems with a great deal of negativity.

Finally, the Water patient has a bluish look to him, a putrid smell and a groaning voice. He is likely to be timid and fearful.

These, of course, are just the bare bones on which the practitioner bases his diagnosis. Among other things, he will also use pulse diagnosis (which I will describe in Chapter Five) to confirm which meridians are affected and in which way they are malfunctioning – that is, whether there is an excess or a deficiency. He may then use a variety of points to stimulate or sedate a meridian or to transfer energy from one element to another.

CHAPTER FOUR

CAUSES OF DISEASE

As we have seen, according to traditional Chinese thinking disease is said to be caused by, among other things, invasion by harmful Chi. We may think of this invasion and the consequent effect that it has on the body in rather the same terms as the Western concept of infection and immunity. If the patient's protecting Chi is lowered, harmful Chi is able to invade and may overwhelm him because his body is unable to fight back. This is similar to the patient whose immune system has been suppressed (for example, by massive doses of steroids following a transplant operation or by an abnormality in the blood such as leukaemia) and who is, therefore, particularly susceptible to infection, against which he has no resistance.

Harmful Chi may also invade, even if the body's protecting Chi is normal, if the former is exceptionally strong. This may be compared to a particularly virulent infection which attacks healthy people whose immune systems are unimpaired. Invasion by harmful Chi in this instance may initially produce an illness but, as long as the invading force is not too strong, the fact that the protecting Chi is normal may allow the body to muster its forces and fight back, as, indeed, it does in so many self-limiting infections. Long-term, chronic illness may be due to a balance between harmful Chi and protecting Chi so that, while the former is not overwhelming, it is too strong for the protecting Chi to fight off entirely.

Disease is not always classified by the Chinese as coming from outside the patient. It can be caused from within and, in this case, may be due to emotional upset, inherited factors or a faulty diet. In the system of acupuncture with which I am most familiar, there are said to be seventeen major factors that cause disease and these are known as the six external factors, the seven emotional factors and the four miscellaneous factors. In addition to these, disease can be due to trauma, poisoning or other physical factors.

It is in terms of these causes of disease that the acupuncturist makes his diagnosis. Unlike a Western physician who will diagnose in terms of which part of the body is diseased and what the abnormality is (for example, inflammation of the appendix, cancer of the lung, cysts in the ovaries and so on), the acupuncturist will make his diagnosis according to what has caused the illness and what effect it has had on the body energies and the function of the zang-fu organs. In this chapter, I will explain the effects that are said to be produced by the different causative factors.

The Six External Factors

The six external factors are associated with weather conditions and may be seen as types of harmful Chi. Because this is essentially a Chinese form of diagnosis, these factors relate to the specific weather conditions prevailing in that part of the world. However, the fact that these were derived in a different climate from our own does not mean that they are invalid in the West, although the frequency of any one type of weather may differ from its frequency in China. These factors are heat, cold, wind, damp, dryness and summer heat. These are all known in the West, although Londoners might be expected to have more illness related to dampness than, say, New Yorkers. The latter, on the other hand, might expect more illness of the summer heat type. In the Far East, too, there are differences in climate. It was mentioned in the first chapter that moxa was used far more in Japan than in China and this was attributed to the fact that Japan has a very humid (damp) climate, moxa being one of the accessory treatments that is used for diseases caused by damp.

When the Chinese talk about invasion by an external factor, what is meant is an invasion by the essential characteristics of that factor, resulting in a disease which reflects those characteristics. In other words, one would not expect a patient who has been invaded by cold necessarily to have a lower temperature than normal, nor does invasion by wind necessarily cause flatulence!

Wind is said to be prevalent in the spring although, in the West, it is perhaps somewhat more common in the autumn. Wind diseases are considered more likely to occur if one is exposed to wind when one is hot or has been sweating profusely or if one has been sleeping in a draught. Wind is predominantly yang in character; it has the attributes of yang, being always moving, insubstantial and agitated, and is often said to attack the upper (yang) part of the body. Headache is a common symptom of diseases caused by wind. Since wind is thought to enter the body through the pores of the skin, it is also thought to disrupt the functioning of the pores, so that the patient sweats excessively.

The patient is not always attacked by wind from outside for it can also develop from within as a result of an excess of yang arising in the liver. The symptoms of internally created wind diseases differ somewhat from those produced by external wind invading the body. In the first case, one might find ringing in the ears and muscle spasms, together with dizziness and headache. In the latter, while dizziness and headache may still occur, the patient may also have a sore throat and a raised temperature.

The characteristics of the external factors are usually related to the symptoms of the diseases that they cause. For example, wind is constantly moving so that diseases which have flitting symptoms are said to be caused by wind. A typical case would be a patient with rheumatic fever. Classically, the patient complains of joint pains lasting, perhaps, no more than a day before they move to another site, and this is combined with fever and sweating. The sweating, as has been mentioned, is related to the wind's effect on the pores of the skin, while the fever relates to the yang qualities of wind, since yang is associated with heat. The patient may also have the headache characteristic of wind-induced diseases and, particularly if the disease has been caused by external wind, he may have a dislike of being in a windy place.

Spasms and twitches of all types, and convulsions, are said to be due to wind, as is facial paralysis, which causes a distortion of the features. This seems rather reminiscent of the English folklore used by mothers who, to stop their children from pulling faces, tell them: 'If the wind changes you'll get stuck like that.'

The external factor of cold is, of course, prevalent in the winter and is more likely to attack someone if he is not warmly dressed or if he is exposed to the cold after getting overheated. Cold is a yin characteristic so, when it invades the body, it overwhelms the body's yang Chi. As a result, an imbalance arises between the body's yin and yang.

The symptoms of disease caused by cold are those which might be expected with an excess of yin – coldness, slowness and inhibition of function. The patient may complain of feeling cold and may shiver. He may look pale. His feet and hands may feel numb or go blue due to poor circulation and he may have cramp in his muscles. Usually, these symptoms are associated with a dislike of the cold. Invasion by cold of the internal organs, particularly the intestines, may cause diarrhoea and abdominal pain. Cold is also associated with stiffness and stagnation, a sort of 'icing up' of the body. The blood and Chi are both liable to stagnate in the presence of cold and the resulting 'accumulation' of either may cause localized pain. Thus, arthritis, in which there is stiffness and localized painful areas, may be due to cold. If this is the cause, the patient may well find that his condition deteriorates during cold weather.

An attack of flu, too, may be ascribed to invasion by cold, if the patient shivers and complains of aching in his muscles. There may be a fever in cold diseases but it is not accompanied by excessive sweating. Frostbite is one condition in which Western medical diagnosis would agree with traditional Chinese medicine that the symptoms of numbness in the feet and hands associated with pallor or blueness were due to invasion of the body by cold.

Like wind, cold may arise internally. With its yin characteristics, cold can develop as a result of a weakening in the yang of the body which thus becomes overwhelmed by yin. A patient who has a cold disease which has arisen internally is more susceptible to external cold than a healthy person, since he has no more yang with which to resist it. If he is invaded by external cold, this will exacerbate his condition and may precipitate a crisis.

Damp in China was said to cause problems mainly in the late summer rainy season. In Japan, as we have seen, it was a far more frequent cause of illness, occurring all the year round. It is a weather condition that we know all too well in Britain! Damp-induced diseases are said to occur after one has had to wear wet clothes for any length of time or if one is constantly in a damp environment. Damp is said to be heavy and stagnant in character and the diseases that are caused by it have similar characteristics, and tend to be long-term problems. The symptoms may include a heavy feeling of the body and the head and the patient may suffer from dizziness. Swelling may occur of the abdomen or of the ankles (known, in Western terms, as fluid retention) and the nose and chest may feel stuffy. Heaviness and chronicity are yin characteristics and therefore damp is predominantly yin. If dampness arises within, it attacks the yang of the spleen and damages it. This can cause chronic digestive problems (since the spleen is considered an important digestive organ). The patient may suffer from recurrent attacks of watery stools or diarrhoea.

In the same way that stagnant water is often polluted and foul smelling, damp, by producing stagnation, is said to cause foul discharges. Foul-smelling and profuse vaginal discharges, smelly, infected urine and oozing skin conditions are all damp-associated.

When damp attacks the upper part of the body, it produces a heavy feeling in the head, a blocked nose, yellowness of the face and difficulty in breathing. These symptoms are not unlike those that might appear, according to Western diagnosis, in a patient suffering from Weil's disease which, interestingly enough, is an infection spread by rats living in or near stagnant water and which is an occupational hazard for sewage workers.

Diseases caused by dryness are associated, in China, with the late autumn – a time that in Europe is more likely to be associated with damp and wind. Dryness, of course, is said to affect the body fluids. In Chinese medicine, as in Western medicine, it is recognized as essential that the body fluids be kept in balance. This balance, in Chinese thinking, is intimately associated with the balance of yin and yang. Dryness itself is primarily yang and therefore can be especially destructive to yin fluid, particularly to the yin fluid of the lung, causing a dry cough, associated with dryness of the mouth and the nose, together with a sore throat.

Dryness may be subdivided into cold dryness and warm dryness. The symptoms of cough and dryness of the throat are common to both, but a patient affected by cold dryness may also have a headache and a dislike of the cold, while a patient whose symptoms are due to warm dryness may be feverish and sweaty.

Naturally, all dry skin conditions, such as certain types of dermatitis, are said to be due to dryness. So, too, are wasting diseases, where the patient looks as though he has been literally dried out, like a prune. Tuberculosis, when it affects the lungs, has the characteristics of dryness, being associated with a dry chesty cough and a general wasting of the body.

Dryness, being yang associated, may also develop internally, owing to a deficiency of yin. However, it may also occur if body fluids are lost through diarrhoea, vomiting or excessive sweating and may thus complicate another disease process.

Heat, naturally, is yang in character and, when it invades, it overwhelms the body's yin Chi, upsetting the natural balance of yin and yang. Summer heat is regarded as a different factor from heat itself, Chinese summer heat being a heavy damp heat. Despite the damp element, the yang component is the strongest and so yang symptoms are still produced. The person who is likely to develop an illness due to invasion by summer heat is one who remains out in the hot sun for a long time or stays in a room with poor ventilation on a very hot day – the kind of conditions that are known by Western doctors to be factors leading to heatstroke.

Summer heat overwhelms the body's yin and injures the body fluids. It may also affect the mind, causing delirium or coma. The onset of the illness may be sudden, since heat is a yang condition and yang is associated with acute onset. Other symptoms of summer heat include profuse sweating and thirst, with a fever and restlessness – all yang characteristics. Heatstroke, as defined in Western terms, shows all these characteristics – thirst, fever and restlessness – and may, also, affect the patient's level of consciousness.

Although heat itself is yang, a patient affected by summer heat may demonstrate yin symptoms if he has been drinking large amounts of cold fluids during the time that he has been exposed to the harmful Chi of summer heat. In such a case, the symptoms would include a feeling of coldness, headache, abdominal pain and vomiting – the sort of symptoms that, in the West, are usually put down to a summer 'tummy bug'.

Heat itself is usually divided into three degrees of severity: fire (the most severe), heat and mild heat. Heat in its most severe form can damage the mind, causing loss of consciousness or coma. It may combine with the other external factors in an invasion of the body, so that some diseases are diagnosed as being due to damp heat, dry heat or to heat and wind. In addition, any of the other five external factors may, if very severe, develop into heat and combine heat symptoms with those of their own.

Many diseases that would be diagnosed by Chinese practitioners as being due to heat would be understood by Western doctors as acute infections, with their common symptoms of fever, thirst and profuse sweating. Local infections, such as boils or abscesses, are also considered to be heat-induced, since they are red, hot and painful. Heat may also cause haemorrhage, since, when it invades the meridians, it is said to drive out the blood that circulates there with the Chi. For example, a patient with a severe intestinal infection who was passing bloody stools would be diagnosed as having had his Large Intestine meridian invaded by heat.

Heat can combine with wind to produce a severe spasm of the muscles and convulsions associated with a high fever. If the patient remains untreated, he may finally become delirious and lapse into a coma. Dryness combined with heat will severely affect the lungs and will cause coughing together with spitting of blood. I said earlier that tuberculosis could be looked upon as being due to an invasion by dryness which produced a dry cough and a wasting of the body. At a later stage of the disease, of course, the patient may start to cough up blood and this would be diagnosed as being due to heat, which developed from the dryness as the latter became increasingly severe. Summer heat may turn into fire, the severest form of heat, and produce an exacerbation of the symptoms that it has caused.

The Seven Emotional Factors

As we have seen, diseases of the type caused by the harmful external factors can, in fact, arise from within the body. Another way in which disease arises from within is as a result of the seven emotional factors which can wear away the body's protective Chi, leaving the patient defenceless. These factors, which are joy, anger, melancholy, obsessional thinking, grief, fear and fright, have to be very intense or very persistent in order to produce disease. When they are this severe, they often damage the internal organs – anger is said to injure the liver, fright and joy the heart, grief and melancholy the lungs, obsessional thinking the spleen, and fear the kidneys. In some books, obsessional thinking is referred to as meditation. However, true meditation and obessional thinking are poles apart and it should not be thought that meditation, as practised by many religions, particularly those of Eastern origin, can harm the spleen, or any other organ!

The emotion of anger has a number of yang attributes such as suddenness, heat, energy of movement and the externalization of the emotions of the angry person, and is, therefore, predominantly yang in character. Its arousal will produce yang symptoms similar to those produced by heat. If the liver, predominantly a yin organ, suffers physical damage as a result of attack by excessive yang, the patient may develop pain and swelling below the right ribs. The liver, in traditional Chinese thought, is responsible for keeping the meridians open and thus allowing an unhindered flow of Chi around the body. It is also thought to be responsible for storing blood. Disruption of its function, therefore, can produce haemorrhage (also, as we have said, associated with heat-induced disease) and menstrual problems. Depression and irritability are also said to result from injury to the liver.

The heart may be damaged by fright – in other words a sudden, severe shock – or by excessive joy. Either can cause the patient to develop palpitations, anxiety, insomnia and mental disorders, since the heart is the seat of the mind. A Western physician, too, would accept that a sudden shock could cause all these symptoms, although it is unlikely that he would agree that anxiety, insomnia and mental problems have anything to do with the heart. He would, however, agree that a heart attack could be precipitated, in a susceptible person, by an extreme shock or, occasionally, even by excessive joy and excitement. Patients with severe angina (chest pain caused by an insufficient supply of blood to the muscles of the heart) are just as likely to develop pain as a result of watching an exciting football match or meeting up with a long-lost friend as they are from becoming angry or upset.

Fright is a sudden, severe, short-term emotion, while fear is more insidious and long term and has to be persistent in order to produce disease. Fear is said to injure the kidneys which are the seat of the will-power. Conversely, if the kidneys are deficient in the functional Chi which is essential for their normal working, the patient is likely to be susceptible to fear.

Injury to the spleen, which is seen as being a part of the digestive system, may occur as a result of obsessional thinking or constant worrying. This may cause anorexia and a feeling of abdominal distension, especially after meals. Obsessional neurosis is a recognized mental state in Western medical terms. Patients suffering from it quite commonly have depression and anorexia as part of their symptom picture. Indeed, anorexia nervosa may be thought of as a form of obsession.

Grief and melancholy (the latter includes anxiety) are said to affect the lungs and therefore may interfere with the breathing. In Western medicine, it is known that anxiety may cause chronic overbreathing, or hyperventilation, and that patients who suffer from panic attacks may be helped to control them by being taught to control their breathing. Anxiety can also be a significant contributory factor in bringing on asthmatic attacks in susceptible patients. When hypnotherapy is used to treat asthmatic patients, one of the ways in which it works is to relieve the anxiety that the patient feels at the onset of an attack and thus to stop the vicious circle in which both anxiety and breathing problems steadily get worse as they feed on each other.

The Four Miscellaneous Factors

As well as the external and the emotional factors, disease may be due to four miscellaneous factors. The first three of these – irregular eating, excessive stress or lack of physical exertion, and trauma – are also acceptable causes of disease in Western medicine, although the symptoms they are said to produce may not be the same. The fourth of the miscellaneous factors is stagnant blood and phlegm.

Irregular eating is a term that includes every form of bad eating habit, such as overeating, undereating, and excessive indulgence in alcohol, fats or spices. It also includes eating food which is going off or has been poisoned, and food which has little nutritional value (the latter being probably more common nowadays in the West, with its 'junk' foods, than in China).

Overeating is said to interfere with the function of the

stomach and the spleen, both of which are intimately concerned in the digestive process. This can cause nausea, vomiting, belching, heartburn, distension, abdominal pain and diarrhoea. Undereating can produce a deficiency in the body's Chi, since food is an important source of Chi, and this will cause weakness, dizziness and emaciation. Unwholesome or poor-quality food will interfere with the function of the stomach and spleen, producing similar symptoms to those caused by overeating. Like Western medicine, Chinese medicine recognizes unwholesome food to be a cause of intestinal parasitic diseases. Excessive indulgence in alcohol, fats and spices will stimulate the production of damp heat within the body which may injure the vital organs. Western doctors would agree that alcohol in excess may damage the liver, while a very fatty diet may damage the heart.

Long-term stress or over-exertion is said to use up the body's protective Chi and thus leave it open to attack by the harmful external factors. It may cause loss of weight, exhaustion, dizziness and palpitations – symptoms that are also associated with excessive stress in the West. However, lack of physical exercise, too, may lower the body's resistance to invasion since it inhibits the flow of Chi and blood around the body and can therefore produce symptoms of weakness, exhaustion, shortness of breath and – as recognized in the West – obesity.

Stagnant blood is said to have left the blood vessels and is therefore no longer circulating around the body. Instead, it is retained in the tissues or in the body cavities and, wherever it accumulates, it causes symptoms. Commonly, it causes pain which may be stabbing or boring in character or, sometimes, colicky (waxing and waning in severity), but the area affected remains constant because the blood is stagnant and therefore does not move. Haemorrhage, either externally or into the skin, and bruising may also be symptoms of stagnant blood. When haemorrhage occurs, it is usually dark in colour and may contain dark clots, unlike haemorrhage caused by heat, which is usually a brighter red. Masses, tumours and swelling of the internal organs may also be caused by stagnant blood.

Phlegm, the partner of stagnant blood in the list of miscellaneous factors, is understood by Westerners to be the sticky fluid that one coughs up from the lungs when one has a chest infection. Although phlegm to the Chinese has the same characteristics, it is not necessarily seen as a sticky fluid and it can affect any part of the body, not just the lungs. It is said to form when the body's use of water is abnormal. Excessive water accumulates within the body and is turned into phlegm which may invade the organs or the meridians. It does not necessarily occur together with stagnant blood, but is lumped together with it in the list of causes because both have stagnant qualities. Like the stuff that many of us have coughed up at one time or another, phlegm is sticky and may completely block the flow of Chi if it invades a meridian. Such a blockage can be the cause of paralysis coupled with numbness, or with difficulty in speaking and distortion of the face, such as may occur in a patient who has had a stroke. Phlegm may, of course, affect the lungs, and cause asthma or a severe cough in which the patient brings up a large amount of sputum. It may affect the stomach, producing abdominal distension and allowing fluid to collect in the abdominal cavity. If it attacks the heart, which is the seat of the spirit, its capacity for causing blockages may result in the patient going into a coma. The rattle that is sometimes heard in the throat of a deeply comatose patient is said to be due to phlegm that is lying there. Various superficial soft, movable lumps which, in Western medicine, might be diagnosed as cysts or lipomata (fat nodules), for example, are said to be due to accumulations of phlegm under the skin.

*

A diagnosis in acupuncture has to be very exact because the more exact it is, the more likely it is that the treatment will be successful. Good treatment is based on good diagnosis. A trained acupuncturist will use the four basic techniques put together by Pien Chueh in the fourth century B.C. – observation, listening and smelling, questioning and pulse diagnosis (this will be covered more fully in the next chapter). Based on this examination he will be able to decide which causative factor is responsible for the illness and how it has affected the body in terms of the meridians and the organs. On the basis of his findings he can differentiate diseases into certain well-defined syndromes (collections of symptoms occurring together). The characteristics associated with individual meridians may indicate which of these are involved in the disease state, and the symptoms may also indicate that certain of the internal, or zang-fu, organs have been affected. The way in which the disease has spread through the body, from one meridian to another, is the province of the Law of the Five Elements, which was covered in the last chapter.

The Eight Syndromes

The syndromes into which diseases may be classified are eight-fold. They consist of four pairs of opposites – exterior and interior, cold and hot, xu (deficiency) and shi (excess), and yin and yang. The four groups are not mutually exclusive, so that one may have, for example, a cold xu syndrome or a hot yang syndrome.

External and internal refer to the position of the disease in the body and, to a certain extent, are related to their severity, since internal diseases are more serious than external diseases. Thus a skin disease or a mild infection such as a head cold would be external, while a disease that attacked the core of the patient's well-being, such as pneumonia, would be internal.

Cold and hot refer to the nature of the disease and the symptoms that these syndromes demonstrate are those that are associated with an invasion of the body by cold or by heat. In a xu (deficiency) syndrome, the protective Chi of the body is deficient and has therefore allowed an invasion by harmful Chi. In a shi (excess) syndrome, however, the protective Chi is normal but it has been overwhelmed by more powerful harmful Chi.

External, hot and shi syndromes, by their nature, are predominantly yang in character, while internal, cold and xu syndromes are predominantly yin. However, it is possible to have cold external syndromes, hot internal syndromes, external xu syndromes, internal shi syndromes, cold shi syndromes and hot xu syndromes, so that, while it is possible to divide all diseases into yin types and yang types, we must always remember that yin and yang are not concrete things but aspects of the balance between two sides of a whole.

Since external syndromes are predominantly yang, they often come on suddenly and are short-lived. Internal syndromes, on the other hand, are more likely to be long term. An external syndrome which is untreated or against which the body cannot defend itself may become more severe and move inwards to become an internal syndrome. For example, an elderly or frail person who catches a head cold which then 'goes onto the chest' and turns into pneumonia may be seen as suffering from an external syndrome which has become internal. An internal syndrome may also be due to an intrinsic disorder of the internal, zang-fu, organs.

Cold syndromes and hot syndromes, as I have said, are associated with the sort of symptoms that are caused by invasion by external cold and heat. Cold syndromes, being predominantly yin, are more likely to be long term than hot syndromes which frequently take the form of acute infections. Xu syndromes, too, being 'empty' and therefore yin, are inclined to be long term, compared with the more acute shi syndromes.

The concept that the internal syndrome is always more serious than the external one is one also found in other complementary therapies, particularly homoeopathy. Hering's Law of Cure is a homoeopathic creed which states that illness is cured from the top down and from the inside out. Thus a homoeopath would say that a patient who has eczema and then develops mild asthma is getting worse, even if his eczema has cleared up. However, a patient with asthma who stops having breathing problems would be said to be getting better, even if he has developed a very severe eczema. The eczema would be seen as the externalizing of his problem, which is an essential step in its cure. Exactly the same is true with acupuncture treatment. A patient who has been suffering from an internal disease may have to trade in his symptoms for those of an external disease before he is finally cured.

In Chinese terms, a common head cold, with its symptoms of running nose, shivering and mild fever, could be classed as a cold external syndrome. However, a diagnosis of a cold internal syndrome would be made on a patient who showed signs of coldness, pale skin, diarrhoea, a high fever and general prostration – symptoms that would be associated, in Western terms too, with a far more serious condition, probably produced by a rampant infection.

A hot external syndrome is associated with symptoms of mild fever and sweating – the sort of thing that one might expect to see in a mild case of flu. In a hot internal syndrome, however, one would find that the patient had a high fever, severe thirst, restlessness, a flushed face, constipation and scanty urine. This is the sort of picture that one might see in a disease such as scarlet fever, a far more serious condition than flu.

Certain types of flu, in which the patient has symptoms of headache and generalized aching in addition to the mild fever, might be diagnosed as external shi syndromes. Internal shi syndromes, however, present the sort of picture that one would associate with pneumonia: a feeling of congestion in the chest associated with difficulty in breathing, malaise and constipation.

Shi syndromes, with their predominantly yang characteristics, are, like external syndromes, usually acute and of sudden onset. They are often associated with fever, flushing of the face and restlessness. The patient may complain of chestiness, abdominal pain or difficulty in passing water, all reflecting the excess or 'full' nature of the complaint. A kidney infection might be classified as a shi syndrome, producing, as it does, fever and abdominal pain of sudden onset, with pain on passing water.

Xu syndromes, which are predominantly yin, are inclined to be long-standing. They are associated with the sort of symptoms that one might expect in a disease where the life force is deficient: listlessness, apathy, poor memory, insomnia, shallow breathing and shortness of breath, poor vision and incontinence, all symptoms that are often found, sadly, in the elderly, chronically ill patient.

Having ascertained the type of syndrome from which his patient is suffering, the acupuncturist then has to decide which parts of the body are primarily affected. This will be based on his knowledge of the meridians and of the zang-fu organs. Symptoms may relate to an individual meridian, particularly when they are localized, and may be associated with the course of the meridian through the body or with the organ to which it is related. (Symptoms associated with the twelve major meridians were mentioned in the previous chapter.)

Certain types of disease are attributed to disruption, by various factors, of the functioning of the vital organs. It may sound as though this localization of diagnosis to a meridian or an organ is akin to the Western practice of diagnosing in terms of a diseased part. However, the difference lies in the fact that acupuncture diagnosis is not saying that a particular meridian or organ is physically diseased, but that its flow of energy has been disrupted in a way that is affecting its function. And this disruption, being one of energy, must therefore have an effect, not just on the organ or meridian itself, but on the whole body.

The Zang-fu Organs

The functions attributed to the organs by Western medicine, such as the heart's role in the circulation of the blood and the kidney's role in the production of urine, are not the only ones recognized by the Chinese. For them, the organs also have other, more subtle, functions in the maintenance of health. The heart, for example, is said to be the seat of the mind, or spirit, and disruption of its function will affect the level of consciousness. Each of the zang ('solid') organs is linked by a channel to a fu ('hollow') organ, and, by another channel, to a sense organ. The heart is linked to the small intestine and to the tongue.

A long illness can result in a general weakness of Chi and this may, in turn, affect the heart. If the Chi, or vital energy, of the heart itself is weak, then this will affect the heart's mechanical function and it may develop irregularities in its beat. As a result, the patient may suffer from palpitations and shortness of breath, especially on exertion, and these are symptoms that the Western physician, too, will associate with heart disease. If the weakness of Chi is not treated, it may develop into a general deficiency of its active aspect, yang, and so result in a total lack of energy, coldness, and pallor (all yin-associated symptoms), together with a susceptibility to other illness.

If the yin of the heart becomes deficient, the symptoms produced may, in turn, be due to the relative excess of yang. In this case, the patient may be restless and feverish and have a flushed face. The deficiency of yin interferes with the function of the heart and thus of the mind, which is housed there, and may cause insomnia or nightmares, poor memory and other mental symptoms. Such symptoms may all occur in a patient who has a high fever.

A long illness may weaken the heart and this, in turn, may interfere with its normal function of pumping blood around the body. A Chinese diagnostician would then say that there was stagnant blood in the heart and that this was the cause of the symptoms and signs demonstrated by the patient: pain in the chest and palpitations, blue lips and blue nails. This corresponds to Western medical thinking to the extent that an orthodox practitioner would recognize these symptoms as being those of an inadequate circulation resulting from poor heart function, although he would not accept the Chinese concept of 'stagnant blood'.

Severe heat, or fire, can also affect the heart. This can arise internally as a result of persistent mental problems which depress the body's Chi and stimulate the production of fire. The symptoms may include fever, reflecting the causative agent, insomnia, due to the effect on the mind which is housed in the heart, and problems affecting the mouth and tongue, such as ulceration, pain and swelling. The latter are due to the fire affecting the parts of the body with which the heart is directly linked.

The functions of the liver are thought to be those of

storing blood, maintaining the flow of Chi around the body and keeping the tendons in good working order. The fu organ to which the liver is linked is the gall bladder (as, indeed, it is anatomically) and Chi runs from the end of the Gall Bladder meridian into the start of the Liver meridian. The sense organ to which the liver is linked is the eye and it is therefore associated with vision and with the maintenance of normal eyesight.

The functional Chi of the liver may become depressed, leading to stagnation of Chi in the Liver meridian. The initial depression of Chi can be as a result of mental problems. If the Chi in the Liver meridian becomes blocked, the patient develops pain below the ribs and in the abdomen, with swelling of the abdomen and, sometimes, of the breasts. Menstrual problems may occur as a result of the stagnant Chi which in turn causes stagnation of blood.

Depression of the Chi of the liver may, in addition, stimulate the production of severe heat, or fire, in the same way as it does when affecting the heart. Fire which affects the liver can also be due to an over-indulgence in alcohol or to excessive smoking. The fire prevents Chi from flowing normally and, as a result, the patient may suffer from dizziness, headache and irritability and develop an inflammation of his eyes. If the blood which is stored by the liver becomes affected by the fire, haemorrhage may result. This can manifest as nosebleeds, or as vomiting of blood.

Heat can be associated with wind in an attack on the liver and, in this case, symptoms are produced that are attributable to both of these external factors. The patient develops a high fever and may have convulsions possibly associated with neck rigidity and, later, coma. These are symptoms recognized in Western medicine as being due to an infection affecting the central nervous system – meningitis or encephalitis.

Cold may affect the liver and cause stagnation of Chi,

particularly in the Liver meridian itself. This causes abdominal pain and, if the patient is a man, can produce swelling and pain in the testicles, since the meridian runs through this area.

The liver is seen as a storehouse for blood, but chronic disease or haemorrhage are said to use up those stores and thus produce a deficiency of blood. As a result, the body is no longer adequately nourished. Other functions of the liver will also be affected: there may be spasm in the tendons and muscles, which depend on the liver for their normal function, and, in addition, the patient may have disturbances of vision, such as blurring and dizziness, and his eyes may feel dry and gritty. If the patient is a woman, her menstrual cycle can be affected and her periods may become scanty and irregular.

The spleen is the organ which is credited by the Chinese with the control of digestion. It is said to be responsible for the proper absorption of nutrients from the ingested food and for their distribution round the body. It also performs the vital function of transforming the Chi that is present in food into a form that can be used by the body, and so is intimately linked with the stomach and its functions. As we saw in Chapter Two, the beginning of the Spleen meridian follows on from the end of the Stomach meridian and receives Chi directly from it. The sense organ to which the spleen is linked is the mouth, although the tongue is associated with the heart. The spleen is also said to control the blood, ensuring that it remains within the blood vessels, and to be responsible for the maintenance of healthy muscles.

As the spleen is involved in the extraction of Chi from food, it will naturally be affected by one's eating habits. Irregular eating habits will cause the functional Chi of the spleen itself to be weakened. Such a weakness may also be due to chronic stress or long-term illness, giving rise to a

poor appetite and inadequate food intake. If the functional
Chi of the spleen is weak, it will be unable to extract Chi
adequately from what little food is being eaten, so that a
vicious circle is set up. The patient develops lassitude, a
sallow complexion and diarrhoea due to the overall deficiency of body nutrition. The muscles are no longer maintained in good condition, so that the body loses its firmness,
and prolapse of the womb or of the rectum (back passage)
may occur. Blood is not properly contained within the
blood vessels and this may result in spontaneous bruising
or haemorrhage.

Because of its intimate association with the stomach and
with digestion, the spleen is susceptible to injury from any
form of unbalanced diet. If excessive amounts of raw or
cold food are eaten, this may lay the spleen open to attack
from cold and damp. Again, this will be associated with
poor appetite and the patient may develop abdominal pain
and diarrhoea. Because cold is inclined to cause stagnation,
the flow of Chi may become blocked and cause swelling in
the upper abdomen, associated with lassitude and a heavy
feeling in the head.

The lungs are, naturally, in charge of respiration which,
in addition to bringing oxygen into the body and expelling
carbon dioxide, takes in clean Chi and gets rid of waste Chi.
In addition, they are said to control the use of water in the
body and to maintain the health of the skin and the hair.
The Lung meridian is coupled in the twenty-four-hour
cycle with one of the other water-controlling meridians, the
Urinary Bladder, so that when one is at its highest point in
terms of the flow of Chi, the other is at its lowest. The lungs
also link with the large intestine (since Chi flows from the
Lung meridian into the Large Intestine meridian) and the
sense organ with which they are connected is, of course, the
nose.

Chronic lung disease from whatever cause may result in a

deficiency of the yin of the lung. This affects the lung's control of the body's water and results in a dry mouth, feverishness, night sweating and a dry cough, sometimes with some blood being coughed up. In Western terms, these are all symptoms associated with a diagnosis of tuberculosis. I mentioned earlier that the symptoms of tuberculosis could be produced by an invasion of the lungs by heat and dryness and, of course, these are both predominantly yang factors whose long-term presence can result in a chronic deficiency of yin.

The lung can also be affected by wind, which may be accompanied by cold. The wind produces a cough and a blocked nose, while the additional cold may aggravate the condition, causing a sensation of coldness, a nasal discharge and the coughing up of sputum. These are symptoms that are often associated with the common cold. If the invading wind is accompanied by heat, the symptoms are those of a rather more severe form of common cold, with fever, a sore throat, and purulent nasal discharge and sputum.

The lung may be affected by the retention within it of damp phlegm or of phlegm. The lung controls the body's use of water but, if this function becomes disrupted, fluid can accumulate to form damp phlegm. This, in turn, blocks the flow of Chi and the patient develops a cough and shortness of breath, and brings up a lot of white sputum. Phlegm may also develop as a result of the invasion of the lung by wind and heat, in which case the symptoms are also due to the effects of heat. Here, too, the flow of Chi is blocked by the phlegm and the patient develops a cough with shortness of breath; in this case, because the phlegm is hot, blood stagnates and, as a result, the sputum that is brought up is not only copious but also purulent.

As well as having a role in the maintenance of the water balance in the body, the kidney is said to be in charge of reproduction, growth and development. Although these last three are not functions associated with the kidney in Western medicine, it is interesting to note that they may be associated with the adrenal glands which are anatomically situated immediately above the kidneys on the back wall of the abdominal cavity. Since the adrenals are the glands that produce the steroid hormones, disruption of their function may produce abnormalities of growth and development and may interfere with normal reproduction. The adrenals also secrete the hormones which regulate the kidney's function of excreting water.

In Chinese medicine, the kidney works together with the lung in its capacity of controlling the body's use of water. The kidney is also said to regulate the distribution of clean Chi, extracted from the inhaled air by the lungs, to the rest of the body. It is responsible for the formation of the bone marrow and blood and also of the brain, which is considered a specialized form of marrow. It is linked to the bladder (as it is anatomically) since the end of the Urinary Bladder meridian opens into the start of the Kidney meridian. The sense organ with which it is associated is the ear, and deafness in the elderly is said to be due to a deficiency of functional Chi in the kidney.

The Chi of the kidney can be weakened by long-term illness or by senility; it is also possible for it to be congenitally weak. Such a weakness will affect urination and can cause frequency, dribbling or incontinence. After a long illness, it may affect the body's reproductive ability and cause infertility. Because of its association with the lung and because of their joint functions, weakness of the functional Chi of the kidney may affect the lung and cause shortness of breath or asthma.

The kidney can also be affected by a deficiency of yin or of yang, either of which may occur as the result of a long illness. Such a deficiency, it is said, may also be due to an over-indulgence in sexual activity. If yin is deficient, the patient may have dizziness, blurring of vision, poor memory and tinnitus (ringing in the ears) due to the kidney's inability to maintain the normal functions of the brain and of the ears. Since a deficiency of yin necessarily results in a relative excess of yang, yang-type symptoms such as feverishness and night sweating will occur.

A deficiency of yang in the kidney will lead to a reduction in the activity of the kidney itself, since yang is associated with activity. This can cause fluid retention and failure to pass adequate amounts of urine. The reduction in activity may also affect bladder function and produce abnormalities such as dribbling and retention of urine. In addition, the relative excess of yin will cause pallor and symptoms of coldness and the patient may become impotent.

As well as being affected through their links with the zang organs, the fu organs can also be specifically affected by a disruption of their own energies. In this case, the position will be reversed and the disruption will also affect the zang organ with which each is associated.

The pericardium may be invaded by heat and this will produce symptoms of high fever, delirium and coma as a result of the effect on the mind, which is housed in the heart.

Jaundice may be diagnosed as an invasion of the gall bladder by damp heat. This may be due to a primary malfunction in the liver or as a result of long-term over-indulgence in alcohol or rich food. Because damp causes stagnation, the flow of Chi is impaired and the resultant blockage prevents bile from being excreted freely. Thus the patient develops jaundice and may vomit bile. It is the blockage of Chi in both the gall bladder and its associated organ, the liver, that produces the pain experienced in the right upper part of the abdomen by many jaundiced patients.

The stomach, like the spleen, will, of course, be affected by an unbalanced diet. Overeating may disrupt its functional Chi, resulting in the retention of food within the stomach. This will cause distension and pain in the upper abdomen, together with belching, nausea and vomiting.

The ingestion of large amounts of raw or cold food may cause the stomach to be attacked by cold. This can also occur if the patient gets soaked by cold rain. The invading cold causes stagnation of the functional Chi of the stomach, resulting in the retention of fluid. This causes the patient to develop pain and swelling in the upper abdomen and, as in the case of the retention of food, he may vomit. Similar symptoms may also be due to depression of the yang of the stomach, which may occur after a long illness. The deficiency of active yang together with a relative excess of yin are the factors that cause the stagnation in this case. Eating large quantities of rich food can cause heat to accumulate in the stomach resulting in a burning pain in the upper abdomen, thirst, vomiting and foul breath.

Although it lies lower down in the digestive tract than the stomach, the large intestine, too, may have its function disrupted by dietary abnormalities. If a person eats excessive amounts of raw or cold food or if he eats food which is unwholesome, the large intestine may be affected by damp heat. The damp causes stagnation and thus hinders the normal flow of Chi. As a result, the patient develops diarrhoea and abdominal pain. The heat may cause haemorrhage and therefore he may pass some blood in his stools. These are symptoms that Western doctors, too, would associate with food poisoning.

Disruption of the flow of Chi in the large intestine may also be due to the stagnation of the blood flow, causing constipation, abdominal pain and distension. A more serious version of this may occur if the stagnation is due to an invasion of the large intestine by heat. This may be due to overeating or a particular susceptibilty of the patient to changes in the weather and, in addition to the symptoms already mentioned, can cause inflammation of the intestine and the formation of abscesses.

Damp heat may invade the bladder and cause the sort of symptoms that are associated in Western medicine with infections of the urinary tract, including frequent passing of water with associated burning and pain. The heat can cause haemorrhage and consequent passage of blood in the urine. If the condition is not treated, the damp may give rise to stagnation which, in turn, may result in the formation of stones.

In the next chapter, we shall look at the methods of diagnosis used by the acupuncturist in deciding the cause of his patient's illness.

CHAPTER FIVE

METHODS OF DIAGNOSIS

Because of his familiarity with the functions of the meridians and of the zang-fu organs, the experienced acupuncturist will usually be able to assess quite quickly which of these has had its flow of Chi disrupted and in what manner. However, to aid him in deciding how this disruption has been brought about he will use pulse and tongue diagnosis. In addition to these, he may look at the patient's face, skin and general appearance and he may ask the patient questions about his eating habits, urine, bowels and sleeping habits. The acupuncturist's findings will help him to determine whether the patient is suffering from a xu (deficiency) syndrome or a shi (excess) syndrome, whether yin or yang is predominant and which of the external, emotional or miscellaneous factors may be responsible for the illness.

The Pulse

Although both Chinese and Western physicians use the same artery – the section of the radial artery that lies at the wrist – when they take a pulse, their methods of doing so are quite dissimilar. Chinese pulse diagnosis is a very exact science, far removed from the simple counting of beats practised in the West, and it may take a student many years of practice before he is proficient at it. Students who have only attended short courses in acupuncture have had no time in which to learn more than the very basics of pulse diagnosis, and will usually rely mainly on the condition of the tongue to back up the diagnosis that they have made based on their knowledge of the meridians and the zang-fu organs. Although tongue diagnosis will give the same indications as pulse diagnosis, it is not nearly so accurate. The difference between a practitioner using tongue diagnosis and one who uses pulse diagnosis as well may be compared to that between two Western doctors, one armed with a stethoscope and blood pressure equipment and one who, in addition, has an ECG (electrocardiogram) machine. The first doctor can quite easily diagnose a patient who has had a heart attack from the symptoms that are presented and from the signs that he can observe with his equipment. However, the doctor with the ECG machine will be able to tell which part of the heart has been affected and how severe the heart attack has been. He will also be able to monitor, on an hour-to-hour basis, any improvement or deterioration in his patient's condition.

When a Western physician takes a pulse, he will put his fingers lightly on one of the patient's wrists and will feel the radial artery somewhere along its superficial course. A Chinese physician, while using the same stretch of the same artery, will feel it at six well-defined places on each wrist, three superficial and three deep. Each of these pulses reflects the condition of one of the twelve major meridians and their associated organs, allowing their balance to be assessed, and the character of the pulse as a whole indicates the type of syndrome which is affecting the patient. Comparing each pulse against the other pulses allows any sign of excess or deficiency in a particular meridian to be detected.

All the superficial pulses are associated with the fu (hollow) organs, which are predominantly yang. On the right are the pulses that are linked to the large intestine, stomach and sanjiao, while on the left are those that are linked to the small intestine, gall bladder and urinary bladder. The deep pulses are associated with the zang (solid) organs, which are predominantly yin: the lung, spleen and pericardium on the right; the heart, liver and kidney on the left.

However, this is not the end of the story where yin and yang are concerned. Left-sidedness is associated with yin and right-sidedness with yang, so all the pulses on the left wrist reflect the total yin of the body and all those on the right wrist the yang. If all the pulses on the right are normal but those on the left are stronger, this indicates an excess of yin, whereas the reverse indicates an excess of yang. Similarly, normal pulses on the right combined with weak pulses on the left suggest a deficiency of yin, while a deficiency of yang would present as normal pulses on the left and weak pulses on the right.

We have already seen that the aspects of yin and yang are not concrete but fluctuate according to how one looks at them and this applies just as much to pulse diagnosis as to anything else. An outer or exterior position is always predominantly yang, compared to an inner position, which is predominantly yin. The outer pulses may be taken to be those that are closest to the wrist and therefore further from the heart, while the inner pulses are those that are slightly higher up the arm and therefore nearer the centre of the circulation. If the outer pulses (relating to large intestine and lung on the right, and small intestine and heart on the left) are stronger than the inner pulses (sanjiao and pericardium on the right and urinary bladder and kidney on the left), this indicates a relative excess of yang in the body. If, however, the inner pulses are stronger than the outer ones, a relative excess of yin would be indicated. The balance of yin and yang may also be determined by comparing the superficial and the deep pulses, since deepness is yin, while superficiality is yang.

Having determined the balance of yin and yang and the balance between the organs and meridians, the acupuncturist will then assess the quality of the pulse in order to elicit further information as to the type of syndrome which is affecting his patient. Numerous qualities of pulse have been described, although many of these categories appear to run into each other and their fine distinctions are perceived only by the expert. However, for our purposes, they may be divided into a few broadly based groups.

The first of these is the rapid pulse which is defined as having more than five beats to a breath (note that in Chinese medicine, the pulse is timed by the patient's breathing and not by the doctor's watch). A rapid pulse often occurs when there is an excess of yang and therefore increased activity in the body or when the patient is suffering from a hot syndrome. This tallies with Western diagnosis, where a rapid pulse (albeit timed by the clock) may be associated with a fever.

This type of pulse may be either forceful or weak, a forceful quality indicating an excess of Chi, or a shi syndrome, whereas a weak pulse would be indicative of a xu (deficiency) syndrome.

Cold syndromes are associated with a slow pulse, also measured according to the patient's breathing. Less than four beats to the breath is taken to be a slow pulse. As with a rapid pulse, a forceful slow pulse suggests a shi syndrome, while a weak slow pulse occurs in a xu syndrome.

The Chinese concept of a normal pulse rate correlates fairly well with that held by physicians in the West, being four to five beats to the breath. In the West, where the pulse is measured as a number of beats per minute, the norm is taken to be around seventy-two, while the normal number of breaths per minute is around sixteen. If one divides the normal pulse rate by the normal breath rate, one gets four and a half, the midway point of the Chinese normal range.

If an excess or a deficiency of Chi occurs without the involvement of cold or heat, as a shi or a xu syndrome, this can also be diagnosed from the pulse. A xu pulse feels weak when pressed lightly and disappears completely on heavy pressure, whereas a shi pulse feels forceful whether one presses lightly or firmly. A thready pulse may also indicate a xu syndrome, while a large bounding pulse may occur in a shi syndrome.

External and internal syndromes also have their own diagnostic types of pulse. External syndromes may be indicated, in the early stage, by a superficial or 'floating' pulse. This is a pulse that is readily felt when the pressure exerted is light but it becomes weak if pressed hard. It gives a sensation of floating on the surface of the skin. A fine distinction of this type of pulse is one which conveys the floating feeling and yet is either weak or forceful. If it is weak, it suggests that the patient is suffering from a long-term illness and a deficiency of yang. A forceful floating pulse, however, would be associated with an external syndrome in which there was an excess of yang.

A deep pulse is diagnostically opposite to a floating pulse. It is necessary to exert increased pressure in order to feel this pulse, which is associated with internal syndromes. Again, it may be forceful or weak, force being associated with an excess and weakness with a deficiency.

Sometimes a pulse is described as being 'slippery' or 'gliding', feeling almost as though it is wriggling under the fingers, and often compared to ball-bearings rolling on a plate. This type of pulse is an indication that phlegm is causing problems and, when forceful, suggests that the seat of these problems is in the digestive tract. If the pulse is weak, however, it suggests that phlegm has accumulated due to a general weakness of the body. A full gliding pulse may occur in healthy people, particularly during pregnancy.

A completely different quality of pulse is referred to as a rough pulse, which has none of the easy movement of the slippery pulse. It may occur in conditions of deficiency of Chi or of blood, particularly if the kidney is affected, in which case it will be weak, or it may indicate stagnation due to an invasion by cold damp, in which case it will be forceful.

An irregular pulse in Western medicine indicates an irregular heart beat due to an electrical misfiring in the mechanism that regulates the contraction of the heart muscle. To a Chinese physician, it is an indication of stagnation of blood with interference to the flow of Chi and a deficiency of yang.

The bowstring or wiry pulse may be found in a healthy person or in one who has a deficiency of yin with a relative excess of yang in the liver. It may also occur in a patient who is in pain and is hard and forceful, giving the impression of a tightly pulled string.

Within these definitions, there are further divisions. For example, as well as the slow and rapid categories, varieties of rate and rhythm may be described as knotted, intermittent, scattered, moving, hasty, slowing or fast.

The Tongue

Tongue diagnosis has fewer nuances than pulse diagnosis and takes less time to learn but is still of great value to the experienced practitioner of Chinese medicine. When he examines the tongue he will look at its colour and condition and also at the colour of its coating. In Western medicine, a healthy tongue is said to be pink and moist and to have little or no coating. This is also accepted as normal in Chinese medicine, but assessment of the tongue goes much further than this and, as with the pulse, the findings are expressed in terms of the cause of the patient's disease and the energy imbalances that have resulted.

A normal tongue is pink, so any obvious variation from this is said to be abnormal. Abnormal colours are classified as pale, red, purplish-red or purple. A pale tongue, as might be guessed, is indicative of a disease caused by cold or of a deficiency syndrome, particularly a deficiency of yang. A deficiency of blood will also cause a pale tongue, and this tallies with the Western inclusion of a pale tongue as one of the signs of anaemia. If the tongue appears glossy and pale, it suggests that the problem is a long-standing one.

If the patient has a wet pale tongue, this indicates that the yang of the spleen is deficient. According to the Law of the Five Elements, the spleen is the master of the kidney. If the spleen is deficient (the paleness indicating deficiency), then it will be unable to control the kidney and this will affect the body fluids, causing the tongue to become abnormally wet.

A red tongue is suggestive of a disease caused by heat or of a deficiency of yin, causing a relative excess of yang. A purplish-red tongue occurs in acute diseases caused by heat, such as acute fevers. In such cases, the tongue may also be dry, indicating that the body fluids have been affected by the heat. A purplish-red tongue can also occur in patients who, due to a prolonged and severe illness, are deficient in yin. In the latter case it is likely to have a glossy appearance, signifying that there has been damage to both the yin and the body fluids.

A purple tongue is one which is recognized by Western doctors as being associated with heart disease, particularly with heart failure and inadequate pumping of the blood round the body. In Chinese medicine, it may indicate a stagnation of Chi and of blood. It may also occur if there is an excess of internal cold, due to a deficiency of yang.

The coating of the tongue is said to be formed from food residues, together with yang Chi derived from the spleen, and thus will clearly reflect any abnormalities of the digestive system. Its colour and condition are also indicative of various states occurring within the body. It may be described as white, yellow, greyish-black or peeled and, in addition, may be thin, thick, sticky, moist or dry. A thick coating usually indicates a more serious problem than a thin coating of the same colour. Patchy coating occurs when the spleen and stomach are not working together as they should in the production of Chi. Moistness is suggestive of invasion by damp, or of an imbalance in the body fluids due to a deficiency of the yang of the kidney or of the spleen, its master according to the Law of the Five Elements. A dry coating is usually due to a deficiency of body fluids as a result of invasion by heat, and a sticky coating suggests that phlegm is the cause of the patient's condition.

A thin white coating may occur in a healthy person but, when seen in a patient suffering from a disease, it indicates an invasion of the lung by wind and cold. A thin yellow coating, on the other hand, is never normal and may indicate an invasion of the lung by wind and heat.

If the coating of the tongue is white and thick, it suggests that food is being retained. A more serious and long-term form of this is suggested by a thick yellow coating.

A sticky white coating indicates invasion of the body by cold and damp or the retention of phlegm and damp in the body. It might be seen, for example, in a patient with bronchitis. A sticky yellow coating indicates retention of damp heat in the body or a blockage in the lung caused by phlegm and heat, and might be seen in a patient suffering from a lung abscess.

A dry white coating to the tongue indicates invasion by a pestilential factor. This is the term used to include all forms of epidemic contagious diseases. A dry yellow coating reflects both heat and an imbalance of body fluids, suggesting an accumulation of heat in the stomach and intestines, which has damaged yin and the associated body fluids.

A yellow coating may, of course, also be seen on the tongues of smokers, so an acupuncturist will always want to know whether or not his patient smokes. His pleasure on finding that a patient is a non-smoker will be two-fold:

firstly, it will make his diagnosis easier; secondly, his treatment will not be counteracted by the patient continuing to assault his body with toxins!

The tongue may sometimes have a bald or peeled appearance. This is often associated, in Western terms, with a severe vitamin deficiency. In Chinese terms, it may indicate a prolonged and severe illness, where the patient's protective Chi has been severely damaged and there is a considerable deficiency of yin – both things that might be associated with malnutrition.

A moist greyish-black coating on the tongue usually suggests that cold and damp have been retained within the body or that inner cold has welled up due to a deficiency of yang and a relative excess of yin. A greyish-black coating that is dry and is seen on a red tongue indicates a drying out of the body fluids by excessive heat which, in turn, may be due to a deficiency of yin with a relative excess of yang. This sort of tongue may occur in patients who, in Western terms, are dehydrated.

The tongue can, of course, be coloured by things other than disease and smoking. Sweets, soft drinks and some fruits and vegetables can all stain the tongue, so it is important to ensure that you haven't dyed it a different shade from your own when you go to see your acupuncturist!

In addition to its colour, the condition of the tongue can reveal important things to the practitioner about his patient's condition. A patient with a large and flabby tongue which is pale and perhaps shows the impression of his teeth around the edge is likely to be suffering from a general deficiency of Chi and of yang and an accumulation within the body of phlegm and of damp. If the tongue is flabby but red, this suggests that there is an excess of heat which is affecting the stomach or the heart. A flabby purplish tongue occurs when there is stagnation of blood. A tongue which is a normal shade of pink may also be flabby and, in this case, it would suggest that there is an accumulation of damp heat in the spleen or in the stomach, or a deficiency of yang.

A tongue which has fissures in it and looks cracked may be normal in some people, so a patient with a tongue like this may be asked whether it has always been like that. If, however, the cracks have only appeared with the onset of the patient's illness, they may indicate a drying up of the body fluids due to excessive heat, and a deficiency of yin, with a relative excess of yang, in the kidney.

The tongue may display little bumps on its surface, which are usually red. These, too, suggest that there is excessive heat with a drying up of body fluids and may also indicate stagnation of the blood. This appearance is called a thorny tongue and it may be seen in a patient who has recently suffered from an infectious illness. White bumps on the tongue or flat purple blotches may occur in severe cases of invasion by heat and the latter may also indicate stagnation of blood and of Chi.

In Western medicine, if the tongue is stiff and tremulous, this is usually associated with some form of neurological disorder. In Chinese medicine, it is an indication of a disturbance of the mind by phlegm and heat. The tongue is, of course, the sense organ that is linked to the heart, which is the seat of the mind. A stiff, tremulous tongue may also be seen in a patient in whom there is a deficiency in the yin of the liver due to an invasion by heat, or may be associated with an obstruction of the collateral channels by wind and phlegm. When it is seen during a prolonged illness, it suggests that there is an overall deficiency of Chi and of yin.

A tongue that is deviated to one side of the mouth, such as may occur after a stroke, is said to indicate obstruction of the collateral channels by wind and phlegm. Wind is often said to be the causative factor of a stroke.

Since wind causes blockages and can therefore interfere

with both movement and sensation, if a patient complains that his tongue feels numb, it may indicate that wind is a causative factor in his illness. This may have arisen either as a result of a deficiency of yin or, if the tongue is red, from an excess of Chi affecting the liver.

A thin tongue is said to indicate a deficiency syndrome. If the tongue is pale, this suggests that the deficiency is one of Chi and of blood whereas, if it is red, the deficiency is likely to be of yin, producing a relative excess of yang.

Tongue diagnosis and pulse diagnosis are the two most valuable methods of diagnosis available to the acupuncturist and this is why I have gone into the details of both techniques before mentioning any others. However, when a patient visits an acupuncturist, it is likely that the other techniques will be used earlier in the consultation: his general appearance will be observed and he will be asked questions about himself before reference is made to his pulse and his tongue.

Patients' Habits

The acupuncturist, like a practitioner of orthodox medicine, may wish to know about a patient's habits, since these may give him some clues as to the problem that is affecting him and as to its cause. Here again, the interpretation that the acupuncturist puts upon the answers that the patient gives will be quite different from that made by a Western physician. For example, a patient who has to stand a great deal in the course of his work may develop problems affecting the kidney and its meridian, while a patient who sits all day may have problems affecting the spleen. The spleen may also be affected by excessive concentration (a lesser degree of the 'meditation' or obsessional thinking mentioned earlier), as may the stomach, with which it works in the digestion of food and extraction of Chi. One may see this sort of effect in the so-called workaholic who spends long hours at his desk, striving for perfection in his work, and finishes up by developing a peptic ulcer.

The patient's eating habits, too, are important, as are his reactions to food. As we have seen, overeating or the consumption of 'junk' foods may contribute towards the development of disease, as may an excessive intake of spices, fats or alcohol. If a patient feels better after he has eaten, this suggests that he is deficient in Chi and that it is the Chi derived from the food he has just eaten that gives him this temporary relief. Conversely, a patient whose symptoms increase in severity after he has eaten has an excess of Chi, with the Chi in the food making matters worse. If he feels bloated after eating, this suggests that the Chi which he has extracted from the food is being prevented from circulating correctly and that there is stagnation. If he is constantly thirsty, this indicates a hot syndrome, while an absence of thirst suggests an invasion by cold or by damp.

Certain tastes are associated with certain of the elements and therefore, when they appear abnormally, may be indicative of problems relating to the organs or meridians associated with those elements. A sour taste is associated with wood, a bitter taste with fire, sweetness with earth, a hot taste (as in curry) with metal and saltiness with water. Thus a salty taste in the mouth may be a symptom of disturbance of the kidney (one of the Water organs) by heat. Since the spleen is associated with earth, damp heat affecting the spleen may produce a sweet taste in the mouth. Heat affecting the fire-associated organ, the heart, is likely to result in a bitter taste. A patient who has lost his sense of taste altogether is likely to have a deficiency of the functional Chi of the spleen. Bad breath is a result of heat in the stomach.

A patient's illness may also be reflected in his sleeping patterns. Excessive sleepiness may be due to a deficiency of yang, with a relative excess of the inactive principle, yin. Insomnia, on the other hand, may indicate a deficiency of yin in the liver and kidney or an overall deficiency of Chi. Early morning waking suggests a deficiency of Chi, particularly in the Gall Bladder meridian, or may be due to an excess of heat in the heart. The heart and gall bladder are also implicated if the patient is a very light sleeper, when a disturbance of the Chi of either may be involved.

Like a Western physician, an acupuncturist may ask the patient about his urine and his bowels, although the conclusions that he draws from the answers that he obtains will be different from the orthodox ones.

If the patient passes a lot of urine or if he has to get up at night to pass water, he has a deficiency in the yang of the kidney. A total deficiency of Chi in the kidney and the bladder, however, may reduce the amount of urine produced to below normal. A deficiency of the functional Chi of the kidney may also produce incontinence.

If there is blood in the urine, it may be an indication of damp heat in the bladder, heat being a common cause of haemorrhage. If the urine is a particularly dark yellow in colour, this also suggests that there has been an invasion by heat, whereas a pale urine indicates an invasion by cold or a deficiency of the yang of the kidney, with a relative excess of yin.

The type of stools that the patient passes may indicate the state of his intestines. Damp, as I have said, is associated with stagnation and foul-smelling discharges. If the patient passes watery, foul-smelling stools, it is a good indication that the intestines have been invaded by damp heat.

While the acupuncturist is interviewing the patient, he will, like any Western physician, be observing him. If the patient appears apprehensive – or perhaps one should say more apprehensive than might be considered normal for a patient on his first visit to an acupuncturist – this may suggest that there is a problem with the kidney or the urinary bladder or with their meridians. If the patient is tense, the liver and gall bladder may be implicated, while a patient whose attention wanders may have problems with the spleen or stomach. The kidney and urinary bladder may also be involved if the patient is overweight or if his hands seem abnormally cold.

A great deal can be discovered by observing the patient's face. As with the tongue, the colour can be very informative. A red face, of course, is suggestive of an invasion by heat. A sallow complexion indicates a deficiency, usually affecting the spleen (which is responsible for the extraction and circulation of Chi) and also suggests an invasion by damp. Damp heat in the spleen may produce a dark, orange-coloured jaundice while a lighter yellow jaundice may be due to damp cold.

A very pale complexion, too, is associated with a deficiency. It may be due to a deficiency of Chi together with cold in the lungs, or it may indicate a total body deficiency of Chi or of yang, such as might occur after a haemorrhage. If the patient's face is pale but his cheeks and lips are red, there may be a deficiency of yin which has resulted in the production of heat through the relative excess of yang.

Pale lips, like a pale complexion, signify a deficiency, particularly in the lungs. Bright red lips, on the other hand, are indicative of heat, especially affecting the heart. Dry lips indicate that heat is affecting the spleen or that there is an imbalance of the body fluids. The condition of the spleen is also implicated if the lips are swollen.

Red and painful eyes may indicate that the patient is suffering from an excess of yang and of heat. If they itch, an invasion by wind and heat may have occurred. The organ with which the eyes are linked is the liver. If the yin of the kidney is deficient and, as a result, it fails to nourish its 'child' of the Five Elements, the liver, the yin of the latter may also become deficient. This may be suspected if a patient complains that light hurts his eyes. A deficiency of Chi in the kidney, resulting in a deficiency in the liver, may produce double vision. Blurred vision, however, can be a result of an abnormality in the blood or of yin.

There are differing views as to the diagnostic value of lines and blemishes in various positions on the face. Some practitioners believe that the entire body is reflected in the face. Others, however, dispute the reliability of this type of diagnosis.

The condition of the skin and the nails is more widely accepted as being of use in diagnosis. Dry, flaky skin suggests that the circulation of Chi and blood is sluggish so that the skin is inadequately nourished. If the skin becomes puffy, this may be due to a blockage in the flow of Chi while a deficiency of Chi will result in the skin becoming thin and wrinkled. If the nails break easily or if they seem soft, this, too, suggests a deficiency of Chi or of blood, particularly affecting the liver upon whose normal function the health of the nails depends.

Although the techniques of acupuncture and the ways in which diagnoses are made are so different from those used in orthodox medicine, a patient who visits an acupuncturist for the first time may well feel, after the initial consultation, that it has been rather similar to that which he might have had with his own family doctor. Many of the questions will have been the same as his doctor might ask, and the examination of tongue, pulse, skin and nails will have a familiar ring to it. And, although the interpretation that the acupuncturist forms from the symptoms and signs presented to him will be very different from the interpretation that would be made by an orthodox doctor, in both Chinese and Western medicine it is on the diagnosis that the treatment will be based.

CHAPTER SIX

METHODS OF TREATMENT

Once he has made his diagnosis, the acupuncturist can decide upon his treatment. As in Western medicine, the treatment will depend upon the diagnosis, but in Chinese medicine the aim of the treatment is not just to get rid of the illness itself but to do this by removing its cause. This is made easier by the fact that a Chinese diagnosis is always couched in terms of the cause of the illness.

In Western medicine both diagnosis and treatment are usually based upon a part of the body – for example, a diagnosis of a broken bone will be followed by treatment of that bone (by putting it in plaster) and a diagnosis of an irregular heart beat will be followed by treatment of the heart (with drugs to regulate its rhythm). A patient diagnosed as having gallstones is likely to have his gall bladder removed and, with it, the stones. However, to remove a patient's gallstones does not treat the initial cause and, although the stones do not re-form, since the gall bladder is no longer there, the imbalance that originally created them has not been cured by the operation. (This imbalance may, of course, be treated by other means, after the operation.)

Chinese medicine bases the diagnosis upon the supposed cause of the illness and treatment is designed to eliminate that cause. A patient whose illness is diagnosed as being due to an invasion by heat, no matter what his symptoms may be, will be given treatment aimed at dispelling heat from the body. Similarly a patient who has an excess of yin will be treated in a way that will sedate yin and stimulate yang. It is possible, sometimes, to treat specific symptoms with acupuncture, since there are some acupuncture points that have specific effects – to lower blood pressure, for example, or to stop vomiting – but these points are not usually used as a complete treatment in themselves.

Acupuncture, like many of the other complementary therapies, is a way of restoring the body's energy flow to a normal state so that the body can get on with the work of healing itself. Therefore when there is a deficiency of Chi, yin or yang, the system must be stimulated, and when there is an excess, this must be reduced. Where there is heat or cold, wind, damp, dryness or phlegm, these must be eliminated from the body, and stagnant blood must be set flowing again. If there are imbalances between the meridians these must be balanced out, by drawing Chi into a deficient meridian from one that has excess. The mother meridian must be encouraged to nourish its child and the master meridian must be adjusted so that it has appropriate control over the servant. If there is a blockage of Chi flowing along the course of a single meridian, this must be unblocked.

On each meridian there are points with specific functions relating to the transfer of energy. The element points have already been mentioned in Chapter Three. In addition, each meridian has a source point by which it is linked to its organ. Thus, the source point on the Lung meridian may be used to treat the lung itself, the source point on the Kidney meridian may be used to treat the kidney, and so on. Some points are specific for dispelling the various external factors: heat, wind, cold, damp, dryness and summer heat. Others have particular effects on yin or yang, either stimulating or sedating. On each of the major meridians, except that of the heart, there is one or more intersection or meridian connection point, with which that meridian is linked to others. These points are useful in treatment of conditions in which the disturbance is affecting several meridians.

Along the Urinary Bladder meridian, as it runs down the back, lie a series of points which have an effect on the other major meridians. These are known as the associated or shu points. Each meridian is related to one associated point lying between Urinary Bladder 13 and Urinary Bladder 28, parallel to the spine. On the front of the trunk are twelve similar alarm or mu points, which are also each connected to one of the major meridians. The alarm points do not lie on a single meridian. Six of them (those relating to the Pericardium, Heart, Stomach, Sanjiao, Small Intestine and Urinary Bladder meridians) are midline and are points on the Ren meridian. The others are bilateral. The Lung alarm point, the Liver alarm point and the Gall Bladder alarm point each lie on their own meridians, but the Kidney alarm point lies on the Gall Bladder meridian, the Spleen alarm point on the Liver meridian and the Large Intestine alarm point on the Stomach meridian. Both the alarm and the associated points may be used diagnostically since, if they become tender or painful, this is an indication of a disturbance involving their associated meridian.

The choice of points to be used in treatment is therefore a very complicated one. The acupuncturist must know the function of each of the points on each of the meridians, plus the non-meridian extra points. He must know how the meridians interact with each other. He must know how to eliminate invasive conditions, such as cold and heat, from the body (certain points on the meridians are specific for drawing off certain types of invasive Chi). He must know how to restore balance to the system and to stimulate it to function normally once more. And, ideally, he must be able to do this all while using a minimum of needles.

At the first lecture that I ever went to on the subject of acupuncture, the speaker projected onto the screen a cartoon which showed a man lying on a couch, stuck full of needles, like a pincushion. The acupuncturist, whom the cartoonist had depicted as Chinese, was standing next to the patient and saying, 'If this doesn't work, nothing will.'

But, as our lecturer observed, what the cartoon really demonstrated was that the person in need of treatment was the acupuncturist!

People are often worried at the thought of being stuck full of needles. But the skill of a trained acupuncturist lies in knowing how to treat a condition using the smallest possible number of acupuncture points. Often a patient may be treated with no more than four or five needles – sometimes a single needle may be enough. If the few points have been correctly chosen then they will produce just as good results as twice as many would. In the next chapter, various illnesses are discussed with diagrams to show which points might be used in treatment. Some of the figures show a considerable number of needles in the 'patient', but an acupuncturist would not use all of these together. Where there is a good choice of equally appropriate points, the practitioner may decide to use only some of them or, in prolonged treatment, may use them all in rotation.

Of course, treatment need not necessarily involve the use of a needle. There are many ways of stimulating the acupuncture points, although needles are probably both the easiest and the most effective, which is why they are the most popular. However, other methods are widely used, both to complement acupuncture and in cases where the use of needles is inappropriate (for example, in the treatment of young children).

Acupressure is the treatment of the acupuncture points by massage. Usually the pressure is 'pulsed' – applied and released a number of times. How long pressure is applied each time may depend on whether or not the point is tender. If it is, the therapist may press for only a second or two before resting. However, the patient will soon realize that, as treatment continues, the point becomes less tender and, after a few minutes, he will be able to stand pressure applied to the point for longer and longer periods. Since a tender acupuncture point is an indication that that point needs treating, the diminution of the tenderness shows that the treatment is working and this can be very encouraging to both patient and therapist.

There are, however, three drawbacks to acupressure. Firstly, only one point can be treated at a time whereas more may be needed, particularly in patients with long-term problems. Secondly, the therapist obviously must be with the patient throughout the treatment, unlike acupuncture where, once the needles are in, the patient may be left for a few minutes while they take effect. Thirdly, the therapist needs to have very strong and resilient hands or he may find that he needs treatment himself – for painful thumbs!

In Chapter One, I mentioned that moxa derives its name from two Japanese words and that Japan used more moxa than China, due to its damp climate. Moxa is still used today to treat conditions caused by cold and damp and, as might be expected, is particularly useful in treating the diseases associated with the damp climate of Great Britain. There are certain points which are particularly susceptible to treatment with moxa.

The usual method of using moxa is to attach a small wad of it to the end of an acupuncture needle which has been inserted into the relevant point. Once the moxa is lit, the warmth it produces travels down the needle and into the point. Since the shortest type of needle commonly in use is an inch long and has a handle which is also an inch long or more, the moxa is never less than about an inch and a half from the skin and therefore the patient is unlikely to get scorched.

Cupping is another method of treating points which need warming in order to eliminate cold or damp. However, unlike moxibustion which is applied to an individual point and can be used on any part of the body, cupping can only be used where there are large flat surfaces, such as the back or the thighs, which are wide enough to take the cup. The cups themselves may be of glass or bamboo and are heated, usually by inserting a burning taper inside them, which creates a partial vacuum. The taper is removed and the cup is immediately placed onto the skin where it adheres by suction, due to the vacuum.

The cups are left on the skin for a few minutes before they are gently prised off, often leaving raised pink marks. These marks usually disappear fairly rapidly. The suction produced by the cups is quite strong (this is what causes the pink marks, since blood is drawn into the surface vessels of the skin) and it is said to draw out the cold or damp which is causing the disease. Cupping is therefore very useful for conditions such as bronchitis where the acupuncturist has diagnosed an invasion by cold or damp and where the actual area affected, that is, the skin overlying the lungs, can be covered by four to six cups. It is also considered effective in moving obstructions, and therefore may be used to treat patients in whom a blockage in the circulation of Chi or of blood has been diagnosed.*

As well as heat and pressure there are many other, less

---

*I have heard it said that the suction produced by cupping can be strong enough to cause a sebaceous cyst to burst, and to draw out all the cheesy matter contained in it. However, it is not a good idea to allow this to happen. It will, temporarily, remove the cyst, of course, but the unfortunate thing about sebaceous cysts is that the cheesy matter is contained within a capsule and, unless this capsule is removed, the cyst will re-form. Since cupping is unable to remove the capsule (this can only be done surgically), the cyst is bound to recur. Not only this, but the breaking of its capsule by cupping (or by any other means) can cause inflammation which can result in it becoming adherent to the surrounding tissues. So it is likely to make its removal by surgery more difficult should you ever wish to have it taken out. If you have a sebaceous cyst, therefore, and you suspect that your acupuncturist is going to use cupping, ask him to avoid putting a cup over the cyst itself. Or, if you prefer, have the cyst removed first, leaving the area free for cupping. Once it has been removed, of course, any acupuncture treatment that you have to restore your body energies to normal should help to prevent you from forming any new cysts.

commonly used, ways of stimulating acupuncture points. These include electrical stimulation, lasers and ultrasound. It is possible that some of the beneficial effects that are achieved by physiotherapists when using ultrasound in the treatment of muscular disorders may be due to the fact that they are, unbeknown to them, treating the correct acupuncture points! However, the commonest form of treatment, and the one that everyone has heard of, is the treatment of points by inserting needles into them.

When people who are not familiar with acupuncture therapy hear about needles being stuck into patients, they invariably think of hypodermic needles, injections and, consequently, pain. And, because of this, many people are unable to understand how it is possible for acupuncture often to be quite painless. But there are two main reasons why injections are painful and neither of these applies to acupuncture. Firstly, because a fluid has to be passed down the hypodermic needle, the needle is hollow. As it enters the skin, it cuts out a tiny section and pushes it into the tissues, causing pain. Then the fluid is injected into the tissues and, as there is no natural cavity there to receive it, it compresses the tissue cells and nerve endings and this, too, is painful. Now, an acupuncture needle is neither hollow, nor is anything forced down it and this is why its insertion feels completely different from having an injection.

Acupuncture needles come in various lengths, ranging from one to three inches, and each has a handle which is another inch or two long. So, at first glance, they may look fairly alarming. However, they are usually only partially inserted into the patient and are only inserted deeply in areas where there is thick muscle, such as the buttocks and thighs. In bony areas, such as the forehead or the hands, only the tip of the needle would be inserted.

The length of time that a needle is left in the patient depends on the practitioner and on the treatment that is being given. Sometimes it is only appropriate to leave a needle in for a second or two. It may be that the purpose of putting the needle in is only to puncture the skin and draw off a drop of blood, creating a passageway through which the body can rid itself of invasive Chi. One practitioner I know, who also practises manipulation, will often insert a needle briefly into a few points around the area that he intends manipulating. This has the effect of loosening the surrounding muscles, making the manipulation easier, and therefore more comfortable, for the patient.

Some practitioners will attach needles to a machine that stimulates them with a mild electrical impulse. This causes the needles to vibrate slightly and produces a mild buzzing sensation. With or without this stimulation, needles may be left in over a period of ten minutes or more. However, once the needles are in, the patient usually feels relaxed and comfortable and does not find the treatment in any way unpleasant. In fact, in the hands of an expert, patients have been known to feel so relaxed that they have dozed off.

Patients may notice that, at different times, the acupuncturist uses different techniques when inserting and removing the needles. This is done according to whether the acupuncturist wants to stimulate the flow of Chi in a case of deficiency, or sedate it in a case of excess. In the former case, he might ask the patient to breathe out as he inserts the needle and to breathe in as he takes it out and, having extracted it, he may massage the acupuncture point into which it was inserted. With a patient suffering from an excess of Chi, the needle might be inserted on an inhalation and removed on an exhalation, and might be rotated while in place. A needle whose function is to stimulate Chi may be inserted so that it lies in the direction of flow of Chi along the meridian while one which aims to reduce Chi might face in the opposite direction.

Ear Acupuncture

Some needles are designed to remain in position semi-permanently. These are the ear studs that are commonly used to help patients who wish to stop smoking or to lose weight. Ear acupuncture was developed in France and is a fairly recent form of treatment, but has become very popular, particularly with smokers who are desperate to give up. It is based on the idea that the human body is reflected, in microcosm, in three parts of itself: the hand, the foot and the ear. Thus, by treating the appropriate part of the hand, foot or ear, the part of the body that it represents can be treated. This is used as the basis of another complementary therapy, reflexology, in which the therapist massages the patient's feet, diagnosing problems by finding areas of tenderness, and treating them by massaging the appropriate points.

In acupuncture the ear is used, in preference to the hand or the foot, but the principle is much the same. A tender area in the ear suggests that the point needs to be treated (as is true elsewhere on the body) and implies that there is an underlying disorder in the part of the body that is associated with that point. Thus, for a patient who is suffering from, say, a sprained ankle, where there is no long-standing disruption of Chi involved, a single needle in the ankle point of the ear may be an appropriate form of treatment. It is particularly useful in the treatment of small children or other patients who do not wish to see the needles going into them.

When using the ear for the treatment of physical disorders there is no need to leave the needles in for longer than the normal period. However, patients who are trying to give up smoking or to diet need continual help and, for them, needles are used that can be left in for about two

weeks at a time. These needles are made of a twist of stainless steel and look very like tiny drawing pins. If a smoker is
being treated, one needle is inserted into the lung point in
the ear. For a dieter, a point in the centre of the area relating to the digestive tract is used. The needle, or stud as it is
sometimes called, is held in by sticking plaster. It may be
slightly painful as it goes in, since the ear is not a very fleshy
area, but this pain should only be temporary and after the
first hour or so the patient should be perfectly comfortable.
Because they have to be held in by tape, ear studs are not
suitable for patients who are allergic to sticking plaster or
for those few patients who develop dermatitis when in prolonged contact with metal. I have known allergic patients,
however, who have been so desperate to give up smoking
that they have taken a course of antihistamine tablets for
the period of time that they needed the stud. A better way
of doing this, perhaps, would be to have a course of acupuncture to try to resolve the allergies before going on to
have an ear stud put in!

Studs are a form of self-help mechanism in that, every
time the patient has a craving for a cigarette (or, in the case
of a dieter, every time he starts to get hungry), he gently
massages the stud with his finger for about ten or twenty
seconds, until the craving, or hunger, disappears. Western
medicine, which likes to find a 'scientific' reason for everything, has discovered that massage of the stud causes the
body to release substances called endorphins into the blood
stream. These are naturally occurring pain-killers, which
the body manufactures and which have an effect not dissimilar to that of morphine (hence the name). They probably do play a role in the action of the stud, but their release
is unlikely to be the whole story since it does not explain
why studs will not work unless they are in exactly the right
place, nor why a stud in the lung point will not help a
dieter, nor one in the digestive tract area a smoker.

Of course, a stud will only help to reduce the physical craving or hunger pangs experienced by the patient. A mental desire to smoke or to eat cannot be damped down by a stud, so the patient must really want to give up smoking or to lose weight. It may sound as though it is just a question of mind over matter, but there is no doubt that patients find that acupuncture studs may work even when they have had no success with plain will-power or with other treatments (including hypnotherapy, which really is a mind-over-matter treatment).

The great advantage of acupuncture studs is that they have no side-effects. Unlike nicotine chewing-gum and appetite suppressants, no drug is entering the patient's system. Therefore they can continue to be used for as long as it takes the patient to achieve his goal. I have known a patient, with a great deal of weight to lose, continue with a stud for over eighteen months during which time she lost weight steadily at around two to three pounds a week – something she had never been able to do before.

Although the treatment is perfectly safe for long-term use, the stud itself must be changed about every two weeks. This is because, even though the studs are sterile and made of stainless steel – and often have a little antibiotic cream smeared on them before insertion – if they stay in the ear for a long time they may act as a focus for infection. So in order to avoid the risk of infection, studs need to be changed regularly. The ear used is alternated in order to reduce the risk still further. Patients are warned that if the stud becomes painful at any time, they should take it out by simply removing the sticking plaster, which will cause the stud to fall out (a point to be remembered by patients who will wash their hair, have showers and even go swimming with a stud in their ears).

CHAPTER SEVEN

HOW ACUPUNCTURE

WORKS: PATIENTS AND

CASE HISTORIES

As we saw in Chapter Five, diagnosis in Chinese terms is quite different from Western diagnosis. And to the Western practitioner, the diagnosis of illness in terms of invasion of the body by wind or by heat may seem bizarre. It must be remembered, however, that this diagnosis is not so much intended to be a literal description of what is actually going on within the body (although sometimes it may be extremely accurate), but rather an indication of what form the treatment should take, since diagnosis and treatment are inextricably linked. When an acupuncturist puts a needle into a point that is specific for dispelling wind from the body, he doesn't expect a rush of air to occur, as though it was being released from a pricked balloon. What he does expect, however, is that when he has diagnosed a disease as being due to invasion by wind, the use of such wind-dispelling points will enable him to improve the patient's condition.

In Western medicine, a single diagnosis does not necessarily mean that there is only one form of treatment available to the patient. For example, a woman who has abnormally heavy periods may be treated with hormone tablets or with a 'scrape' of the womb. A patient suffering from depression may be offered antidepressant tablets, electro-convulsive therapy or psychotherapy. A patient with a duodenal ulcer may have it treated with medication or by operation. Often it may be left to the patient to decide which form of treatment he would like to try first. But in acupuncture, treatment is far more clear-cut. If a patient has a disease which has been caused by invasion by heat, then the treatment is to rid him of the excessive heat, to balance out any consequent imbalance of yin and yang and to restore the flow of Chi to normal.

For a patient in whom injury has caused a blockage of the normal flow of Chi (for example, a patient with a sprained ankle) and where the resulting pain is diagnosed as being due to blockage of Chi or to stagnant blood, the treatment is to release the block or disperse the blood. Naturally, this all sounds very unscientific, as well it might when one remembers that these are the descriptions that have been used for over two thousand years. However, it is the indication that these descriptions give us as to treatment that is important. And since, when used by an expert, the diagnosis and the treatment that automatically follows on from it can produce remarkably beneficial results, it seems unimportant that the diagnosis is couched in terms that have no relevance to modern Western medicine as we know it.

In this chapter, I want to look at some disorders that are commonly diagnosed in Western medical practice and see how an acupuncturist might diagnose and treat them. However, since in life things are seldom as simple as they seem to be in the textbooks, I will also include, at the end, some actual case histories from practice.

Arthritis

Since acupuncture is usually associated in people's minds with the idea of the relief of pain, arthritis is probably one of the most common complaints for which patients, initially, go to an acupuncturist.

In Western terms, we are able to divide arthritis into two broad categories: osteoarthritis and rheumatoid arthritis.

Osteoarthritis is a disease that results from wear and tear and therefore it occurs more commonly in older patients. If it occurs in younger people, it has usually developed in a joint that has previously been damaged. It affects mainly the large joints, particularly the hip which has spent a lifetime carrying the body around. Deposits of calcium are laid down in the joint whose natural surfaces have been worn away, and the patient finds that the joint becomes stiff and causes pain, especially on movement. Rheumatoid arthritis, on the other hand, is an inflammatory condition and can affect people of any age, including children (when it occurs in young children it is known as Still's disease). On the whole, it attacks the smaller joints which become inflamed and distorted. Some patients recover completely, while others may be left crippled, but the majority of people who suffer from rheumatoid arthritis have a certain degree of disability without it ever becoming very severe. For some reason, this condition is much more common in women than in men.

The main feature of both types of arthritis is that the joints are painful and stiff and may be swollen. Chinese diagnosis sees these symptoms as being due to a blockage of the flow of Chi, either because the meridians affected have been invaded by external harmful Chi, or because a meridian has been damaged by injury.

Damage to a meridian may, at first, remain quite localized but, if untreated, the disruption to the flow of Chi may spread and affect other meridians. For example, if a footballer is kicked on the side of his knee, it can become bruised and swollen. This may then resolve so that his knee returns to normal. On the other hand, if he tries to play football while it is still recovering, this could interfere with healing and the joint might become more painful until the condition is chronic. A Western physician would say that the initial blow had set up a reaction within the joint which, aggravated by further stress, had resulted in the development of an arthritic condition. A Chinese physician might say that the initial blow had disrupted the flow of Chi in the Gall Bladder meridian which runs down the side of the knee, and that, because the flow had not been allowed to return to normal, the disruption had spread to involve the Urinary Bladder meridian, running down the back of the leg, the Stomach meridian, running down the front of the leg, and then the Liver, Kidney and Spleen meridians so that there was a circle running round the knee through which the flow of Chi was blocked.

It is the blockage of Chi that causes the pain and the swelling. The acupuncturist's treatment will attempt to relieve the block and disperse any invasive Chi which may have been the precipitating cause. However, arthritis often occurs in more than just one joint and our footballer is not the typical arthritic patient.

Let us take the imaginary case of a middle-aged woman who comes to see the acupuncturist complaining of pain in her joints which she has had for some years. The pain has gradually been getting worse and she finds that it is particularly bad if the weather is wet or cold. It is, to some extent, relieved by warmth and she finds that she is more mobile in the summer months. The pain in her wrists and the numbness and pain in her fingers make it increasingly difficult for her to do housework, to sew or to write a letter.

Two important points in this history are that the condition is chronic and that it is made worse by cold and damp. It would seem, therefore, that cold and damp may be the external factors involved (both of these being liable to produce chronic conditions). The conditions that, in the West, are diagnosed as rheumatoid arthritis, rheumatic fever, gout, and other problems that present with painful joints, are commonly known in Chinese diagnosis as bi syndromes. Bi implies an obstruction – both to the flow of Chi and to the blood. Thus, in this woman's case, it would seem that she has a bi syndrome caused by an invasion by cold and damp.

On examination of this patient, she is found to have some swelling around the affected joints and this, too, suggests that there is an obstruction to the flow of Chi. Her tongue has a thin, moist, white coating which, in a patient who is unwell, indicates an invasion by cold and damp. Finally, her pulse is deep and slow which indicates that the condition is internal – and therefore chronic – and cold in nature.

To treat this patient, one would use points that would disperse the invading cold and damp and remove the obstruction to the flow of Chi. Because of the chronicity of the condition, the body's production of protective Chi also needs to be stimulated, to help her to fight back. And one could also treat specific areas, such as the wrists and hands, that were particularly troublesome. Moxibustion, with its effect of warming the acupuncture points, would be particularly useful in counteracting the invasive cold and damp.

Figure 16 shows the points that might be used, together with their Chinese names and their meridian number (the meanings of their names are given in the text). It is important to note that the diagrams in this chapter show only the approximate positions of the points mentioned and not their exact locations.

Hegu (whose name means 'valley of harmony') is used to disperse cold from the body; it also unblocks obstructed meridians and sets Chi flowing again. Zusanli (whose name means 'three houses') affects both the blood and the Chi, returning them to normal. Qihai (meaning 'sea of Chi') adjusts the flow of Chi to normal. Both Zusanli and Qihai strengthen the entire body. Moxibustion is used on Xuehai ('sea of blood') to disperse cold from the body; this point,

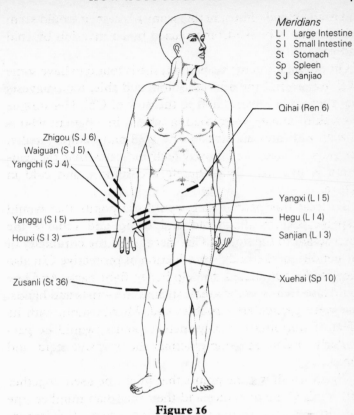

Meridians
L I Large Intestine
S I Small Intestine
St Stomach
Sp Spleen
S J Sanjiao

Qihai (Ren 6)

Zhigou (S J 6)
Waiguan (S J 5)
Yangchi (S J 4)

Yangxi (L I 5)
Hegu (L I 4)

Yanggu (S I 5)
Houxi (S I 3)

Sanjian (L I 3)

Xuehai (Sp 10)

Zusanli (St 36)

Figure 16

as might be guessed from its name, also stimulates the blood. Zhigou ('branch ditch') encourages the circulation of Chi around the body and disperses stagnant blood. Yangchi ('pool of yang'), Waiguan ('outer gateway'), Yangxi ('stream of yang') and Yanggu ('valley of yang') are all used for their local effects on the wrist joint. In addition, Yangchi and Waiguan will unblock obstructed Chi. Similarly Houxi ('tributary rivulet') and Sanjian ('third space') have a local effect on the fingers.

Thus the effect of all these needles would be to unblock

obstructed meridians, to clear out invading cold and to stimulate the circulation of blood and of Chi around the body.

Now let's look at a patient who, in Western terms, has an acute attack of rheumatoid arthritis. The interesting thing here is that both this patient and the middle-aged woman just described might be treated by an orthodox practitioner with the same sort of drugs – anti-inflammatory preparations or possibly even steroids. However, if one is using acupuncture, the two patients are treated quite differently from each other because the diagnosis is no longer the same in both cases.

Let us assume that this second patient is a thirty-year-old woman who has recently developed swelling and pain in several of her joints. She has a mild fever and the affected joints are red and feel hot to the touch. The pain in her joints is not constant, as it was with the other woman; some days her knees are the most painful, on other days it's her wrists, and sometimes it's her feet that are the most troublesome.

Listening to her story, the acupuncturist will decide that there has been an invasion by heat (causing the redness of the joints and the fever) and by wind (causing the flitting character of the pain from one joint to another). Looking at her, he sees that her face is flushed which, again, indicates the presence of a hot disease. Her tongue is red and has a yellow coating and her pulse is rapid and forceful. All of these confirm the diagnosis of an invasion by heat.

So, in this case, the treatment is to dispel the heat and the wind and, if necessary, to treat local painful areas. The points that might be used are shown in Figure 17. Dazhui ('great club') and Quchi ('crooked pool') both have the effect of cooling heat and expelling wind from the meridians. Zhigou stimulates the circulation of Chi and disperses stagnant blood. Liangqiu ('main hill'), Dubi ('nose of the calf'), Yanglingquan ('yang monument foun-

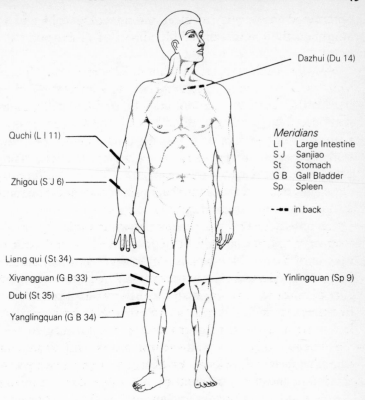

Dazhui (Du 14)

Quchi (L I 11)

Meridians
L I Large Intestine
S J Sanjiao
St Stomach
G B Gall Bladder
Sp Spleen

Zhigou (S J 6)

- ■ in back

Liang qui (St 34)
Xiyangguan (G B 33)
Dubi (St 35)
Yanglingquan (G B 34)

Yinlingquan (Sp 9)

Figure 17

tain'), Xiyangguan ('yang gateway') and Yinlingquan ('yin monument fountain') are all useful for their local effect on the knee joint (this is assuming that on the day that she is seen by the acupuncturist, these are the joints that are causing our patient the most trouble). In addition, Liangqiu stimulates the circulation of Chi, while Yanglingquan has a cooling effect on heat.

Here again, the overall effect of treatment is to dispel the causative factors – in this case, wind and heat – and to unblock obstructions to the flow of Chi. Once Chi is flowing normally and the heat has been dispersed, there will no longer be anything in the patient's body that can cause the joints to swell or to be painful.

Migraine

This is another complaint that often finds its way into the acupuncturist's clinic, since it is a problem that Western medicine cannot always treat successfully.

The generally accepted medical theory of migraine is that it is caused by an abnormal spasm, followed by an abnormal dilation, of the arteries in the brain, specifically of those supplying the front part of the brain. The initial spasm results in insufficient blood flowing to the eyes and this is the reason why many patients have visual symptoms – flashing lights or even total blindness – at the start of a migraine. Then the arteries relax and dilate so that an abnormally large amount of blood reaches the area that so recently has been deprived. It is this great surge of blood that causes the severe headache. Usually, once a migraine has developed, ordinary pain-killers such as aspirin and paracetamol will have little effect on it. Western medical treatment is aimed at trying to stop the migraine before it gets to this stage by preventing the arteries from behaving in this abnormal way. The ergot derivatives which form the basis of a number of migraine treatments are vaso-constrictors – in other words, they prevent the over-dilation of the arteries and thus stop the headache from developing.

Let us now look at a young woman who comes to the acupuncture clinic complaining of recurrent migraine. She describes the pain as running from just above one eye, across the top of her head and down into her neck. It is severe and throbbing and her face becomes hot and flushed.

And let us say that, on her way to keep her appointment,

the patient starts to develop a migraine, so that by the time she sees the acupuncturist, the headache is beginning to develop quite strongly. Looking at her, the acupuncturist sees that her face is red, indicating a hot condition. When he examines her eyes, they appear inflamed and she complains that the light hurts them. This suggests that the heat is a result of an excess of yang. Her tongue is red and has a yellow coating which, again, signifies heat. Her pulse is rapid, due to the heat, and both forceful and floating in character, which indicates an external syndrome with an excess of yang.

The treatment of this patient, therefore, would be aimed at reducing this overabundance of yang and bringing yin and yang back into balance. This will then cool the heat which has arisen as a result of the excess of yang. The path that is taken by the pain – running from the eye, across the head and into the neck – corresponds to the route of the Gall Bladder meridian in this part of the body, a meridian often disturbed in patients with migraine. The acupuncturist may feel along the course of the meridian for tender points which will need treatment – one acupuncture teacher I know delightfully calls them the 'ouch' points, but their correct Chinese name is the ah-shi (meaning 'oh, yes!') points. These points will probably be tender even when the patient feels well if she has been suffering from recurrent migraine.

Treatment may be given either during the migraine itself, in order to stop the attack, or between attacks when the patient feels well. In either case, the balancing out of yin and yang should help to prevent further attacks. The patient may be advised to stop smoking, drinking and eating red meats, since these are factors that may stimulate the formation of excess yang.

Figure 18 shows the points that might be used in the treatment of this patient. The points along the Gall Bladder

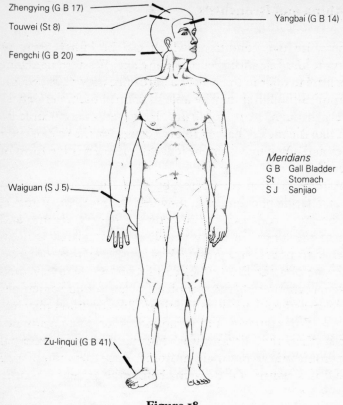

Figure 18

meridian – Yangbai ('white yang'), Zhengying ('exact plan') and Fengchi ('wind pool') – are the supposed ah-shi points for this hypothetical patient. Touwei ('angle of the head') is a specific point for the treatment of migraine, as is Zu-linqui ('foot above tears'). Waiguan has an effect on all the yang of the body and is able to bring it into balance with yin; in this case, therefore, it would reduce the excess.

Asthma and Bronchitis

These are two conditions which can be either acute or chronic and can affect people of any age. Western medicine has little to offer in the way of a cure once they have become chronic although it may be able to control them very effectively through the use of drugs. However, many people do not like the idea of having to take drugs for the rest of their lives and some may start to look for an alternative form of therapy.

Asthma is often considered by Western practitioners to be an allergic phenomenon, in which the bronchi, or tubes, of the lungs constrict and impede the flow of air into and out of the lungs. In many people it is associated with an allergy to pollen and an attack of hay fever may progress into one of asthma. In other cases, children who have had eczema (another allergic problem) when young sometimes develop asthma later on while their skin condition may improve. This course would be an indication to an acupuncturist that the disease was turning from an external syndrome into an internal syndrome. Treatment might well result in a return of the eczema before the patient was fully recovered.

In many cases of allergic asthma, the allergen, or substance to which the patient is allergic, is house dust. Other common allergens are feathers and animal fur, so that budgerigars, cats, dogs and horses will set off an attack if they come near the patient. Asthma also has a psychological component: because it is a very frightening condition, the fear that arises when an attack starts may of itself make the attack worse, thus forming a vicious circle.

Asthma may be associated with bronchitis in an individual patient, but they can occur independently of each other. Bronchitis is an inflammatory condition of the bronchi (or 'tubes') brought on by anything that causes the lungs to become inflamed, such as infection and smoking. An acute attack, which presents as a bad cough accompanied by the production of large amounts of yellow or green phlegm, and which is due to a bacterial infection, may be completely cured by treatment with antibiotics. However, a series of attacks can cause permanent damage to the lungs, especially if the patient is a smoker, which will prevent the bronchitis from ever resolving completely, or if the attacks are inadequately treated, or if there is another contributory condition present, such as asthma. If this is the case, the patient may go on to develop chronic bronchitis, with a permanent productive cough and shortness of breath – a condition which is commonly seen in patients who have smoked heavily for years.

Let us take as an example, first of all, a patient who would be diagnosed by a Western physician as having asthma. He is a young man who, periodically, develops a tight feeling in his chest which makes it difficult for him to breathe. During these attacks he wheezes and coughs up some white frothy sputum. If he gets upset, this may bring on an attack. On examination, he is found to have a sticky white coating on his tongue and a slow pulse that feels like a taut wire. From these symptoms and signs, the acupuncturist can diagnose that the patient has congestion in his lungs which is due to invasion by cold (because the pulse is slow) and by phlegm (because of the sputum and the appearance of the tongue). This congestion is caused by spasm (indicated by the bowstring pulse) and is therefore interrupting the normal flow of Chi. This type of asthma is also said to be brought on by exposure to a cold wind when the patient is tired and may be made worse by emotion.

Treatment of this patient would entail using points to disperse the cold and the phlegm, and using moxa or cupping to warm the lungs. A number of points might be used, some of which are shown in Figure 19. Fengmen ('gate of

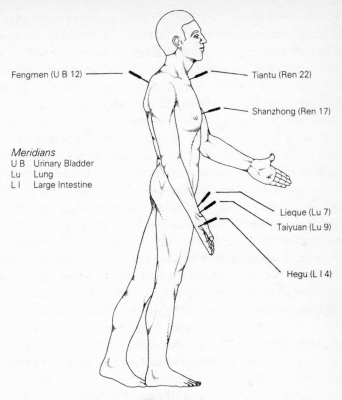

Fengmen (U B 12) ———

Tiantu (Ren 22)

Shanzhong (Ren 17)

Meridians
U B   Urinary Bladder
Lu   Lung
L I   Large Intestine

Lieque (Lu 7)
Taiyuan (Lu 9)

Hegu (L I 4)

Figure 19

the wind'), Tiantu ('heaven rushing') and Shanzhong ('centre of altar') relieve congestion in the lungs and stimulate the circulation of Chi, and are special points for use in the treatment of asthma. Taiyuan ('great abyss') disperses phlegm and Lieque ('distinct depression') and Hegu dispel cold from the body.

In orthodox practice, this patient would be treated with a drug which would cause the spasm in the bronchi to relax, as would our next hypothetical patient, who would also receive an antibiotic. This second patient is somewhat older than the first, being in his fifties, but he presents with the same tight feeling in his chest and wheezy breathing. In addition, he has a slight fever and a chesty cough. The spasm in his chest prevents him from coughing up very much sputum but that which does come up is thick and either yellow or green. On examination, his pulse is fast and is slippery or gliding in quality. His tongue is red and has a sticky yellow coating. The diagnosis here is one of invasion of the lung by heat which has caused stagnation of Chi and the formation of phlegm. This is indicated by the fever, fast pulse and red tongue with yellow coating, all of which signify heat, and by the slippery pulse, the sputum and the stickiness of the tongue coating which all signify the presence of phlegm.

Again, a number of acupuncture points may be used in treatment, some of which are shown in Figure 20. Feishu ('lung shu, or associated, point'), Kongzui ('most excellent') and Chize ('fertile area') all disperse heat from the lungs and stimulate the functional Chi of the lung. Fenglong ('great abundance') removes phlegm and Tiantu stimulates the circulation of Chi in the lung and is a special point for the treatment of asthma.

Finally, on the topic of asthma, let us look at a child who has chronic asthma and who, in orthodox medicine, would be treated in a similar way to the two patients already mentioned. This little boy, let us say, is eight years old and has had asthma since the age of three. The recurrent attacks have interfered with his normal development and he is underweight and short for his age. He gets tired easily and is inclined to be restless. On examination, his face has a yellowish tinge to it and his lips are pale. His tongue looks pale and has a thin, white, sticky coating; his pulse feels forceless and disappears on pressure. The characteristics of his pulse plus the colour of his face and lips suggest that this is

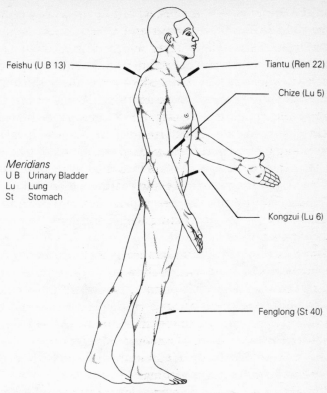

Feishu (U B 13)

Tiantu (Ren 22)

Chize (Lu 5)

Meridians
U B Urinary Bladder
Lu Lung
St Stomach

Kongzui (Lu 6)

Fenglong (St 40)

Figure 20

a xu, or deficiency, condition. This is also suggested by the general condition of the boy, that is, small and underweight. His pale tongue, too, indicates a deficiency, while its sticky white coating points to an invasion by cold, damp or phlegm. The deficiency has obviously affected the lungs, producing the symptoms of asthma, but, since the kidney is the organ that is in charge of growth and development, it would seem that there is a deficiency there as well. According to the Law of the Five Elements, the Lung meridian,

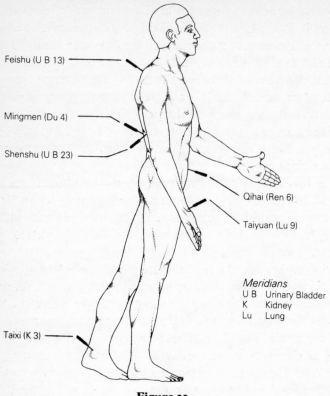

Feishu (U B 13)

Mingmen (Du 4)

Shenshu (U B 23)

Qihai (Ren 6)

Taiyuan (Lu 9)

Meridians
U B   Urinary Bladder
K   Kidney
Lu   Lung

Taixi (K 3)

Figure 21

being metal, is mother to the Kidney meridian, which is, of course, water. Thus a deficiency in one may, if long term, easily affect the other.

A possible treatment of this patient is shown in Figure 21. Obviously, a long-term problem such as his would need a long course of treatment, and the points used would probably vary from session to session depending on how his condition was reacting. The functional Chi of the kidney is stimulated by Shenshu ('kidney shu point'), Mingmen ('gate of command'), Qihai and Taixi ('large rivulet').

Feishu removes blockages in the lung and stimulates the circulation of Chi. Taiyuan is the source point for the lung, which means that it forms a direct link with the lung and can be used to stimulate it. It can also be used in connection with the Law of the Five Elements. The Lung is the yin Metal meridian, and it is the child of the Spleen meridian, which is the yin Earth meridian. Taiyuan is the Earth point of the Lung meridian and therefore can be used to stimulate the yin Earth meridian. Thus the mother is stimulated to nourish the child.

It has already been said that asthma and bronchitis can exist independently, so finally in this section let us bring into our imaginary acupuncture clinic two patients suffering from bronchitis – one with the acute condition, the other with the chronic.

Let us say that the first of these patients became ill a week or so ago when he developed a head cold, with a running nose, fever and a general feeling of being unwell. Since then, he has started to cough and is bringing up quantities of thick yellow sputum. This is the type of complaint that is regularly seen in the general practitioner's surgery in Britain during the winter months and is usually treated with a course of antibiotics. On examining our patient, the acupuncturist finds that he has a rapid pulse, a flushed face and a red tongue which has a thin yellow coating. All this points to a diagnosis of an invasion by heat, the thin yellow coating on the tongue suggesting that wind may also be involved. If wind invades the lung and blocks the circulation of Chi, phlegm will form, and the fact that the patient has been coughing up sputum is another indication that this is what has happened.

Figure 22 shows some of the points that might be used in treating this patient. Heat is dispersed by needling of Feishu and Dazhui while wind is eliminated by the use of Lieque and Hegu and both are dispersed by Quchi.

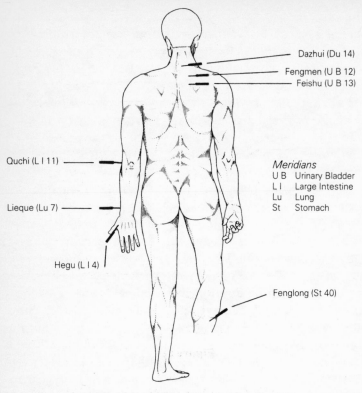

Dazhui (Du 14)
Fengmen (U B 12)
Feishu (U B 13)

Quchi (L I 11)

Meridians
U B   Urinary Bladder
L I   Large Intestine
Lu   Lung
St   Stomach

Lieque (Lu 7)

Hegu (L I 4)

Fenglong (St 40)

Figure 22

Fenglong and Fengmen eliminate phlegm and the latter also stimulates the flow of Chi in the lungs.

The treatment of our chronic bronchitic patient is somewhat different. He complains of a constant cough which becomes worse in winter, lack of appetite and lack of energy. Western medicine applies the term bronchitis to him as well as to the last patient because both are seen as having inflammation ('itis') of the tubes of the lungs. However, in Chinese medicine there is always a fundamental difference between acute and chronic conditions since acute

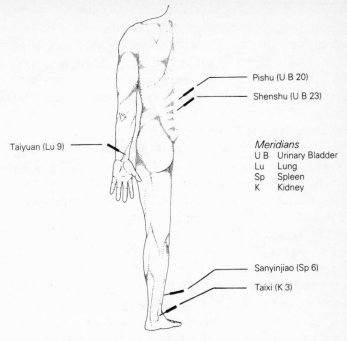

Taiyuan (Lu 9)

Pishu (U B 20)
Shenshu (U B 23)

Meridians
U B   Urinary Bladder
Lu   Lung
Sp   Spleen
K   Kidney

Sanyinjiao (Sp 6)
Taixi (K 3)

Figure 23

implies external and often hot syndromes, possibly with an excess of yang, while chronic suggests internal, cold and excessively yin syndromes. When the acupuncturist examines this patient who has chronic bronchitis, he finds that he has a pale tongue with a sticky white coating and a deep, slow pulse. His pale tongue and deep slow pulse, together with his symptoms of lack of appetite and energy, suggest that this is a xu (deficiency) syndrome. The sticky white coating on the patient's tongue indicates that cold and damp or phlegm are factors in the causation of the disease. Thus treatment would be aimed at stimulating the energy of the lungs and dispelling the cold and phlegm.

Figure 23 shows the points that might be used to treat

this patient. Pishu ('spleen shu, or associated, point'), Taiyuan and Sanyinjiao ('three yin channels', an intersection point for the Spleen, Liver and Kidney meridians) can be used to disperse phlegm. The first two also stimulate the Earth meridians. Thus the Spleen meridian is stimulated to nourish its child, the Lung meridian. Shenshu and Taixi stimulate the kidney. This is of use since the Kidney meridian is the yin Water meridian and thus the child of the Lung meridian. Stimulation of its functional Chi will prevent any deficiency in that meridian from contributing to the deficiency in the lung. Naturally, a patient with chronic bronchitis will need a much longer course of treatment than one with acute bronchitis in order to obtain relief from his symptoms.

Gall Bladder Disease

This is not a problem that one might immediately think of taking to an acupuncturist for treatment since in orthodox practice it is usually dealt with surgically. Western physicians divide it into two main types: cholecystitis (inflammation of the gall bladder) and cholelithiasis (gallstones). Very often, the two may occur together. Both are painful conditions and commonly occur in women around the age of forty, the patients frequently being overweight. Cholecystitis often has an acute onset, with the patient complaining of a severe pain just under the base of the rib cage on the right-hand side. The pain is constant and the patient may become feverish and may vomit. Usually the cause is an infection, sometimes due to the fact that there are stones in the gall bladder, and its orthodox treatment would consist of antibiotics in the acute stage, followed by the removal of the gall bladder at a later stage when the infection had settled down. When uncomplicated by infection, gallstones are more likely to be associated with a colicky, or spasmodic, pain due to the gall bladder trying to squeeze the stone out or to a stone actually passing down the bile duct leading from the gall bladder to the small intestine. However, the symptoms of the two complaints may be very similar and it may be necessary to take X-rays in order to establish whether or not there are gallstones present. A gall bladder that contains stones, whether or not it is causing symptoms, is usually removed complete with stones.

With either cholecystitis or gallstones the patient may vomit and, if the flow of bile into the small intestine is blocked, by inflammation or by a stone, jaundice will develop.

In order to see how such a patient might be treated by acupuncture, let us imagine that an acupuncturist is called to see a thirty-nine-year-old woman who is complaining of a severe pain under the right side of the rib cage, with fever and jaundice. On examination, her tongue is found to be red and to have a sticky yellow coating and her pulse is rapid and forceful. The situation of the pain indicates a problem with the liver and gall bladder which lie together under the right-hand border of the rib cage. Jaundice is usually interpreted to be an indication of an invasion by damp heat. This is corroborated by the appearance of her tongue and the fever. The forceful quality of the patient's pulse suggests a shi (excess) syndrome and the involvement of heat further suggests that this is an excess of yang.

Some points that may be used are shown in Figure 24. Yanglingquan, Ganshu ('liver shu point') and Danshu ('gall bladder shu point') have the action of eliminating damp heat and stimulating the circulation of Chi in the Liver and Gall Bladder meridians. Zhiyang ('very yang') dispels damp and brings Chi back into balance. Xingjian ('walking between') reduces heat in the liver and mobilizes Chi which has become stuck. It is also the Fire point of the

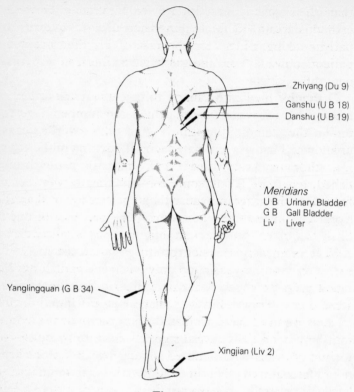

Figure 24

meridian. Fire is the child of wood, and the Liver and Gall Bladder are Wood meridians. In a shi syndrome it is customary to treat the child, while in a xu syndrome one treats the mother.

Hypertension (High Blood Pressure)

This is a problem which can be controlled very well by modern drugs so that the majority of patients suffering from it probably would not think of looking any further than their general practitioner for treatment. However, orthodox treatment for hypertension usually involves the patient taking tablets for the rest of his life, and some patients nowadays are not too keen on the idea of permanent pill-taking.

Orthodox medicine cannot fully explain the cause of most cases of hypertension, which are lumped together under the name 'idiopathic' – in other words, cause unknown. That it is associated with hardening of the arteries, atheroma, heart disease and strokes is firmly established, but there is still some confusion as to what comes first: does the atheroma cause the hypertension or does the hypertension cause the atheroma? The presence of one is likely to worsen the other and thus create a vicious circle.

Very often, hypertension produces no symptoms in its early stages and is picked up only when the patient has his blood pressure checked during a medical examination for some other reason. However, diagnoses in Chinese medicine, as we have seen, are based upon the patient's symptoms and upon the outward signs, backed up by pulse and tongue observations. A raised blood pressure, as such, is not a recognized sign in traditional Chinese medicine because, naturally, when acupuncture was first developing thousands of years ago, there was no equipment for measuring blood pressure. However, if a patient, whose blood pressure has been found to be raised on testing but who has no symptoms, goes to an acupuncturist, examination of his tongue and pulse (plus the other signs used by practitioners of the Five Elements school) should indicate a diagnosis in Chinese medical terms. And his treatment will then be based on this.

Let us consider, as an example, a patient who has already developed symptoms from her hypertension. She is an elderly lady, rather frail, who is complaining of slight dizziness, blurred vision and recurring headaches. She also has difficulty in sleeping and wakes early in the morning. Her face is pale but she has pink cheeks. Her tongue is red and slightly glossy in appearance, and she has a weak and rapid pulse.

Hypertension is said to be due to either an excess of yang or an excess of phlegm and damp. In this lady's case the former would seem to be the cause, being secondary to a deficiency of yin. Such a deficiency may occur in the liver or kidney (which control the circulation of Chi) simply as a result of growing old. A deficiency in the kidney will result in its child, the liver, becoming undernourished. Hyper-activity of the yang of the liver, due to a deficiency of yin with which to balance it, may produce dizziness. Head-aches, a red tongue and a rapid pulse also indicate an excess of yang (producing an inner heat), while a coexisting defi-ciency of yin is suggested by the blurred vision, sleeping problems, glossy tongue and weakness of the pulse. Blurred vision is particularly associated with a deficiency in the liver which is linked to the eye. A pale face with pink cheeks is indicative of a yin deficiency which is causing a relative excess of yang.

This lady may be helped by treatment using some of the points shown in Figure 25. Taixi stimulates yin and sedates yang and, like Sanyinjiao and Shenshu, stimulates the function of the kidney. Xingjian is usually used together with Taichong ('great rushing') in the control of blood pressure, since the latter stimulates yin and sedates yang while the former reduces heat in the liver.

If hypertension is caused by an invasion of phlegm and damp, the picture is quite different. We may imagine, in this case, a middle-aged man who, like the previous patient, complains of dizziness but, unlike her, is not frail but over-weight. He also suffers from palpitations and occasional chest pain. On examination, he is found to have a slow and

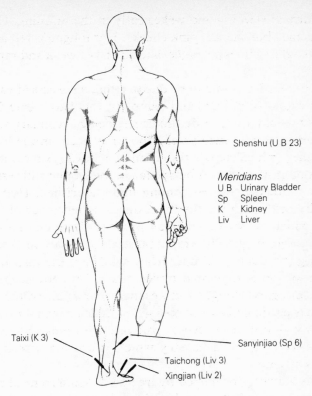

Shenshu (U B 23)

Meridians
U B   Urinary Bladder
Sp   Spleen
K   Kidney
Liv   Liver

Taixi (K 3)

Sanyinjiao (Sp 6)

Taichong (Liv 3)

Xingjian (Liv 2)

Figure 25

deep pulse and his tongue has a sticky coat. Because it is related to eating habits, obesity is said to have a damaging effect on the spleen which distils Chi from the ingested food. As a result, the formation and circulation of Chi is affected. The sticky coating on his tongue suggests that phlegm and damp have developed in conjunction with the poor circulation of Chi. The deep slow pulse indicates an internal syndrome and corroborates the findings on the tongue.

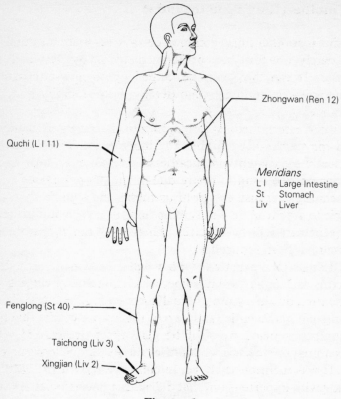

Zhongwan (Ren 12)

Quchi (L I 11)

Meridians
L I   Large Intestine
St   Stomach
Liv   Liver

Fenglong (St 40)

Taichong (Liv 3)

Xingjian (Liv 2)

Figure 26

Retention of phlegm and damp within the body causes mental clouding and would be the reason for this patient's dizziness. His treatment would consist of clearing out the phlegm and thus returning the function of the spleen to normal. The points that might be used are shown in Figure 26. Fenglong and Quchi expel phlegm, Xingjian mobilizes Chi which has become obstructed and Taichong and Zhongwan ('centre channel') are specific points for treating hypertension.

Tinnitus (Ringing in the Ears)

This is another fairly common chronic problem but, unfortunately, one for which orthodox medicine has very little to offer. It can, however, be helped by various alternative therapies, including hypnotherapy, homoeopathy and, of course, acupuncture.

In Western medical terms, tinnitus is caused by damage to the nerve that supplies the inner ear and is therefore usually associated with deafness. The patient's hearing is poor on two counts: firstly due to the nerve damage and, secondly, because the tinnitus masks the sounds that are able to get through. Thus, if the tinnitus can be diminished, the patient will hear better, whether or not the deafness itself has been reduced.

Let us take a patient with what is known in orthodox terms as Ménière's syndrome, which consists of ringing in the ears, dizziness and gradually worsening deafness. He is a man in his seventies and he tells the acupuncturist that his tinnitus is made worse if he gets upset or stressed. On examination he has a weak pulse and his tongue looks pale.

It was mentioned above, in connection with the elderly lady with hypertension, that old age may be associated with reduced functioning of the kidney and a reduction in its functional Chi. The sense organ with which the kidney is linked is the ear, so a deficiency of Chi occurring in the elderly as a chronic condition may have an effect on the ear, reducing its functioning, and causing deafness. The patient's deep, weak pulse and his pale tongue, together with the fact that his symptoms are aggravated by stress, all suggest the presence of a xu syndrome. The dizziness is due to a deficiency in the brain (or 'sea of marrow') whose maintenance is dependent on the normal functioning of the kidney.

In treatment, the aim is to strengthen the kidney and to

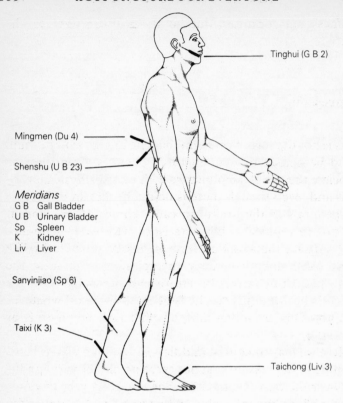

Tinghui (G B 2)

Mingmen (Du 4)

Shenshu (U B 23)

Meridians
G B   Gall Bladder
U B   Urinary Bladder
Sp   Spleen
K   Kidney
Liv   Liver

Sanyinjiao (Sp 6)

Taixi (K 3)

Taichong (Liv 3)

Figure 27

reinforce its functional Chi. This may be done by using some of the points shown in Figure 27. Shenshu strengthens the Chi of the kidney, as do Mingmen and Taixi. Taichong reinforces the yin element of the kidney and liver while Sanyinjiao strengthens the kidney and stimulates the liver. Here again, the treatment is based on the relationship between the Kidney (Water) and Liver (Wood) meridians in which the former is the mother of the latter and a deficiency in one will, if long continued, affect the other. Tinghui ('hearing ability') is a specific point for deafness and tinnitus, due to its position next to the ear.

Depression

This is not the sort of problem that one might, at first, think could be helped by acupuncture. There is a tendency to associate the use of acupuncture with purely physical problems and, even though there is no doubt that an imbalance of chemicals in the brain can cause clinical depression, it has no truly physical characteristics. However, acupuncture can have remarkable effects on mental states since, like many other complementary therapies, it is treating the whole patient by raising his entire level of health. Thus if a patient's health improves, he is likely to shake off whatever symptoms are troubling him, whether they be physical or mental.

Here we may imagine a middle-aged woman who is complaining of depression that has crept up on her very gradually over the past few months. She also feels very anxious, often without knowing why – a common accompaniment to depression. She has difficulty in sleeping and has the typical early morning waking so often experienced by the depressed patient, waking at around five in the morning and unable to get to sleep again. She also has occasional bouts of dizziness and feels totally devoid of energy all the time. On examination, her face is pale and her skin looks dull. Her tongue appears flabby and there are indentations around its edge, made by her teeth. Her pulse is slow and disappears on pressure. These findings, together with her symptoms, all point to a deficiency syndrome. Since the heart is the seat of the mind, it would seem that her deficiency of Chi has affected the Heart meridian. Treatment would there-

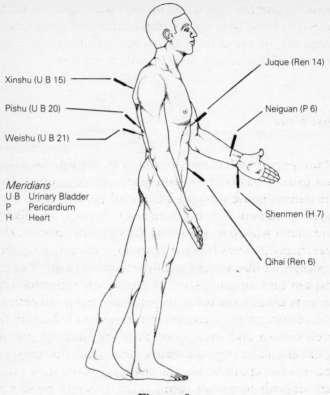

Xinshu (U B 15)

Pishu (U B 20)

Weishu (U B 21)

Meridians
U B   Urinary Bladder
P   Pericardium
H   Heart

Juque (Ren 14)

Neiguan (P 6)

Shenmen (H 7)

Qihai (Ren 6)

Figure 28

fore be aimed at stimulating the production and circulation of Chi and ensuring adequate nourishment of the heart.

Figure 28 shows some of the points that might be used for treating this woman. Shenmen ('gate of the spirit') is a specific point for depression and is the most important point for balancing the energies of the heart. This is also achieved by using Xinshu ('Heart shu point'), Juque ('great shrine') and Neiguan ('inner gateway'). In addition, Xinshu and Juque, together with Qihai, strengthen Chi and stimulate its circulation. Pishu and Weishu ('Stomach shu point') stimulate the action of the spleen and the stomach which are the two organs responsible for extracting Chi from the ingested food and whose malfunction may be responsible for diminished Chi within the body.

Insomnia

Many people suffer from insomnia at one time or another and usually this is just a temporary problem, often due to the patient going through a stressful period. If he is prepared to wait until the problem resolves itself, he is likely to find that it will do so as soon as the stress has passed. However, many patients become so anxious about their inability to sleep that this anxiety itself contributes to the insomnia, and can turn an acute state into a chronic problem. These patients usually see their doctors and obtain sleeping tablets, often with the intention of taking the medication for a week or two and then, once they are sleeping normally again, gradually stopping taking them. Unfortunately, once one is on sleeping tablets, no matter how mild, it may be very difficult to get off them, since the body rapidly gets used to them and, although the patient may sleep very well while taking tablets, without them he may suffer from an insomnia that is worse than it was before he started.

Very often, patients will seek the advice of an alternative therapist not at the onset of the insomnia, but after they have been on sleeping tablets for some time and have experienced difficulty in coming off them. Some acupuncturists maintain that the effects of sleeping tablets (and other tranquillizers) on the system to some extent counteract the effect of acupuncture, so they will ask patients to come off their tablets even before they start to have treatment. And because the drugs are still in the patient's body, it may be a little while before the treatment starts to work. However, if he perseveres, the patient will find that acupuncture not only helps him to sleep, but will also speed up the excretion of the sleeping tablets from his body. Other acupuncturists will treat the patient while he is still taking tablets and will allow him to come off them, in his own time, once he begins to feel the effects of the treatment.

Let us take, as our example here, a middle-aged man who has found it increasingly difficult to sleep over the past few months. When he does manage to get to sleep, he dreams a great deal. He says that as a result of his sleeplessness he is becoming very irritable, he gets dizzy and has an intermittent ringing in his ears. He is also getting pain in his back, which he puts down to his tossing and turning at night. On examination, his face is pale but his lips are red, his eyes look dull and his tongue is red and thin. His pulse is rapid and disappears on pressure.

From the fact that this condition is affecting the patient's mind (with sleeplessness, dreaming and irritability), we can determine that his heart, the seat of the mind, has been affected. The irritability, red lips and rapid pulse are all indicative of heat. However, his other symptoms, pale face and disappearing pulse, speak of a deficiency. Dullness of the eyes suggests a deficiency of yin in the kidney. As we saw previously, in the case of the elderly lady with hypertension, hyperactivity of the yang of the liver, due to inadequate nourishment of yin by the kidney, can produce dizziness. A red thin tongue is indicative of a deficiency of yin producing internal heat due to the relative excess of yang.

The meridian which has, so to speak, got out of control in this way is the Heart meridian. In the servant–master relationship, the Heart meridian is the servant of the Kidney meridian and so a deficiency in the latter could produce symptoms of overactivity or heat in the former. Treatment

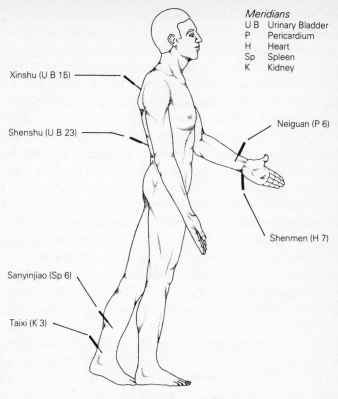

Xinshu (U B 15)

Shenshu (U B 23)

Sanyinjiao (Sp 6)

Taixi (K 3)

Meridians
U B   Urinary Bladder
P   Pericardium
H   Heart
Sp   Spleen
K   Kidney

Neiguan (P 6)

Shenmen (H 7)

Figure 29

will therefore have to stimulate the function of the kidney while sedating the activity of the heart.

Figure 29 shows some of the points that might be used to achieve this. Shenmen is the source point of the Heart meridian and is therefore the one that connects directly with the heart itself. Use of this will calm the heart and restore it to normality. Neiguan and Xinshu will also calm the heart and the latter balances the functional Chi of the heart. The Chi of the kidney is strengthened by Sanyinjiao, Taixi and Shenshu.

Facial Paralysis

This is a condition which is known in Western medicine as Bell's palsy. The region of the face that is affected is that supplied by the facial nerve which, for reasons unknown, becomes suddenly inflamed and swollen. Only one side of the face is affected, other nerves are not involved and the condition is limited to the face. Eighty-five per cent of patients with Bell's palsy recover completely, but recovery can be a long process, taking nine months or more before the nerve is working normally again.

Let us suppose that a forty-five-year-old man has come to the acupuncture clinic, showing the usual signs of this condition: an inability to shut the eye on the affected side (let us say, the left) completely, watering of that eye, drooping of the left corner of his mouth and a paralysis of the muscles that makes it impossible for him to do anything with the left side of his face, such as smile, frown or whistle. On examination, the left side of his face appears slightly swollen, as does the area around his left eye. His tongue has a white coating and his pulse is superficial in character and slow. As with all patients suffering from this condition, he says that it came on rapidly, over the course of a day or two.

In Chinese medicine, paralysis of any type is said to be due to a complete blockage of the flow of Chi and of blood. The suddenness of the onset of this attack suggests that it was due to an invasion by wind. This diagnosis is also suggested by the puffiness of the patient's face and eye. The white coating on his tongue and his slow pulse indicate that cold has also been a factor in producing the obstruction to Chi. The aim of treatment, therefore, is to disperse the wind and the cold and to stimulate the circulation of blood and of Chi. Moxa may be used to warm the points.

Figure 30 shows a selection of the many points that may be used in this condition. Wind may be eliminated by treat-

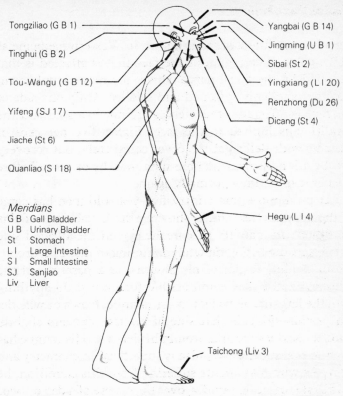

Tongziliao (G B 1)

Tinghui (G B 2)

Tou-Wangu (G B 12)

Yifeng (SJ 17)

Jiache (St 6)

Quanliao (S I 18)

Yangbai (G B 14)

Jingming (U B 1)

Sibai (St 2)

Yingxiang (L I 20)

Renzhong (Du 26)

Dicang (St 4)

Hegu (L I 4)

Meridians
G B Gall Bladder
U B Urinary Bladder
St   Stomach
L I   Large Intestine
S I   Small Intestine
SJ   Sanjiao
Liv Liver

Taichong (Liv 3)

Figure 30

ment of Hegu, Taichong, Tinghui and Tou-Wangu ('complete bone'). Yifeng ('wind screen') relieves any local pain. It is also a powerful point for the elimination of wind and the breaking down of the obstruction to the flow of Chi and blood. Elimination of wind and breaking down of the obstruction may also be produced by Dicang ('storehouse of earth'). Jiache ('cart of the jaws'), Quanliao ('cheek bone'), Jingming ('bright eyes'), Tongziliao ('orbit bone'), Sibai ('four whites'), Yingxiang ('fragrant meeting') and Renzhong ('centre of man') all have a similar action. Yangbai is used to unblock the obstruction and to strengthen blood and Chi. Naturally, only some of these points, perhaps three or four, would be used at the same time and the treatment would be changed, if necessary, as the patient progressed.

Heatstroke

This condition used to be called sunstroke, and English people who lived in the tropics would never go out of doors without a hat on, in order to avoid the supposed evil effects of the sun on their heads. However, it is not the sunshine itself but the heat that it produces that causes the condition, particularly when the atmosphere is very humid and the patient cannot therefore rid himself of heat by the evaporation of sweat. Here, Western medicine is in agreement with Chinese medicine which gives the cause of heatstroke as invasion by summer heat, which is a fierce, damp heat.

If we picture a patient with this condition, he is flushed, thirsty and has a headache. His mouth is dry and his pulse is superficial and bounding in character, and rapid. He is slightly confused.

The signs all point to invasion by heat and the confusion suggests that the heart (the seat of the mind) has been affected. The treatment is to disperse the heat affecting the body.

Some of the points that might be used are shown in Figure 31. Pricking Weizhong ('sustaining centre') in order to make it bleed is a specific treatment to expel summer heat. Heat is also dispersed by treatment of Hegu, Quchi and Dazhui, while Daling ('big monument') acts specifically to reduce the heat affecting the heart.

Gastroenteritis

Our patient in this case may also be one who has been visit-

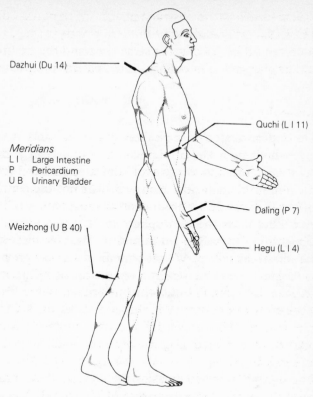

Dazhui (Du 14)

Quchi (L I 11)

Meridians
L I   Large Intestine
P   Pericardium
U B   Urinary Bladder

Weizhong (U B 40)

Daling (P 7)

Hegu (L I 4)

Figure 31

ing a hot country. Many people find that they are unable to take a holiday in a hot climate without developing a holiday 'tummy bug', and a number of medications are available over the counter in chemists' shops that are specifically advertised as helpful in combating holiday tummy.

Let us say that this patient is a young man who is having a two-week holiday in Spain. After a couple of days out there, he has developed abdominal pain and is passing hot, yellow, loose and smelly stools which burn his anus as he passes them. He has a slight fever and is sweating. He has vomited a couple of times and, although not feeling able to eat, he keeps drinking water as he is thirsty most of the time. He has a sweet taste in his mouth which the water does not wash away. On examination, his face is flushed and his lips are dry, despite the continual sips of water. His tongue is red and has a sticky yellow coating and his pulse is rapid with a slippery, or gliding, feel to it.

The passage of smelly, loose, yellow stools is indicative of an invasion of the spleen, stomach and intestines by damp heat. The normal extraction of Chi from food by the stomach and spleen is disrupted and the circulation of Chi becomes disordered; it is this that causes the vomiting. The fever and thirst, together with the patient's flushed face and red tongue, confirm the involvement of heat. A sweet taste in the mouth suggests heat and damp in the spleen while dry lips are also indicative of heat in the spleen. A rapid pulse, of course, signifies heat, while its forceful, slippery quality implies an invasion of the digestive tract by damp which is blocking the digestive process. Treatment aims at eliminating the damp heat and restoring the stomach, spleen and intestines to normal working order.

Figure 32 shows some of the points that may be used in treating this patient. Damp heat in the intestines can be eliminated by the use of Neiting ('within the house'), Hegu and Yinlingquan. The latter also strengthens the lower jiao (the lower abdominal cavity and its contents) and, together with Neiting, Tianshu ('axis of heaven'), Zusanli and Dachangshu ('large intestine shu point'), unblocks obstructions affecting the intestines. Neiguan stimulates the circulation of Chi; this helps to prevent vomiting by stopping the abnormal movement of Chi. Zhongwan is also a specific point for treating vomiting since it stimulates the circulation of Chi and brings the functional Chi of the stomach back into normal balance.

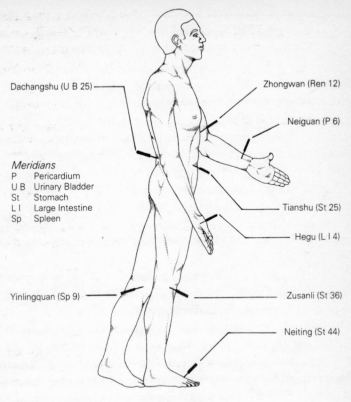

Dachangshu (U B 25)

Zhongwan (Ren 12)

Neiguan (P 6)

Meridians
P   Pericardium
U B   Urinary Bladder
St   Stomach
L I   Large Intestine
Sp   Spleen

Tianshu (St 25)

Hegu (L I 4)

Yinlingquan (Sp 9)

Zusanli (St 36)

Neiting (St 44)

Figure 32

Bedwetting

All children who wet the bed grow out of the habit eventually, but some take longer than others. When the condition continues beyond the age of three or four, it can be a great nuisance, not only to the parents who have to change the sheets but also to the child who may become very anxious about his inability to stop. There are various orthodox treatments available. The 'buzzer' is an electronic device which is sensitive to damp and, as soon as the child starts to wet the bed, the buzzer goes off and wakes him up. Some children find this very effective. Another common treatment is the use of imipramine, a drug which is frequently used in adults as an antidepressant. This, too, is effective but naturally there are parents who do not wish their children to take drugs unless it is absolutely unavoidable. Of course, some children respond to neither of these treatments and require an alternative form of therapy to help them to stop bedwetting. For them, acupuncture may prove to be very useful.

In Chinese medicine, bedwetting is seen as a lack of control over the urine due to a deficiency in the Water (Kidney and Urinary Bladder) meridians, and treatment is aimed at strengthening these.

Figure 33 shows some of the points that could be used for this treatment. The functional Chi of the kidney is strengthened by Shenshu , Guanyuan ('main gateway') and Qihai and that of the bladder by Pangguangshu ('bladder shu point'), while Zhongji ('central pole') helps to restore normal function to both. Obstruction to the flow of Chi is removed by Sanyinjiao, which also strengthens the kidney, and Dadun ('very generous').

Impotence

This is another condition in which the kidney is involved. In Chinese medicine, the kidney is thought to be responsible for governing the reproductive system and so any abnormalities in the patient's sexual function are said to stem from problems relating to the kidney. Since impotence may be seen as a form of deficiency, with aspects of internalization and lack of movement, the element that seems to be deficient would be yang, resulting in a relative excess of yin.

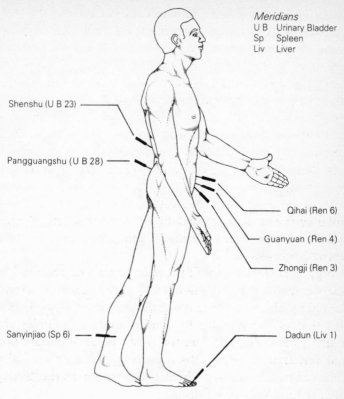

Meridians
U B   Urinary Bladder
Sp   Spleen
Liv   Liver

Shenshu (U B 23)

Pangguangshu (U B 28)

Qihai (Ren 6)

Guanyuan (Ren 4)

Zhongji (Ren 3)

Sanyinjiao (Sp 6)

Dadun (Liv 1)

Figure 33

The deficiency may involve not only the Kidney meridian but also the Ren meridian (or Vessel of Conception) which is the midline channel running down the front of the body. The Ren meridian is associated with the sexual organs because of its pathway. Treatment of impotence consists primarily of stimulation of the yang of the kidney in order to restore balance.

Possible points for use in treatment are shown in Figure 34. The yang of the kidney is strengthened by Mingmen, Shenshu and Taixi. Guanyuan is a major point for

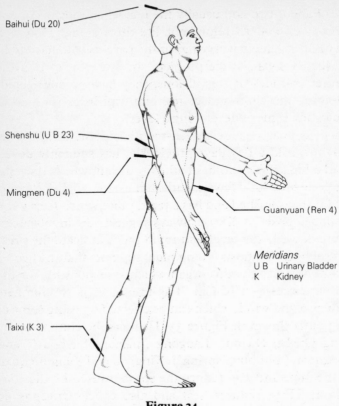

Baihui (Du 20)

Shenshu (U B 23)

Mingmen (Du 4)

Guanyuan (Ren 4)

Meridians
U B   Urinary Bladder
K   Kidney

Taixi (K 3)

Figure 34

strengthening yang and Baihui ('many abilities') has a similar action. Moxa may help the effect by warming the meridians.

Febrile Convulsions

Certain children are prone to have fits if they develop infections that cause their temperatures to rise rapidly. Fortunately, it is a susceptibility that most grow out of after the age of about two and usually the fits, when they occur, are short-lived and therefore not life-threatening. However, they are extremely worrying for the parents who have to be constantly aware of the problem. In order to try to avoid further episodes of convulsions, they have to start tepid-sponging the child and giving him aspirin as soon as he shows any signs of developing a fever.

Let us imagine an eighteen-month-old girl who, having caught a cold a few days previously, has suddenly developed a high fever and has had a fit, during which time she has gone blue for a few seconds. On examination following the fit, she is flushed and has a rapid pulse which feels wiry. A sudden onset of disease always suggests the involvement of wind, while the fever and rapid pulse indicate the presence of heat. Cyanosis (going blue) suggests that the liver is involved, since it is this organ which is responsible for the normal circulation of Chi. The treatment is to eliminate both heat and wind, which can be effected by using some of the points shown in Figure 35. Heat can be eliminated by using Quchi, Dazhui, Laogong ('palace of labour') and Yongquan ('bubbling spring'). Xingjian and Yanglingquan do the same and also reduce the spasm caused by the convulsion. Hegu reduces heat and also expels wind, as do Shangyang ('yang consultant') and Shaoze ('lesser marsh'). Taichong expels wind from the liver and is a specific point for the treatment of fits. Kunlun ('mountain in Tibet') expels wind from the head and clears any residual mental clouding, as does Houxi. Renzhong is a major point for resuscitating patients whose whole system has undergone a shock.

Urticaria

In Western medicine, urticaria is seen as an allergic

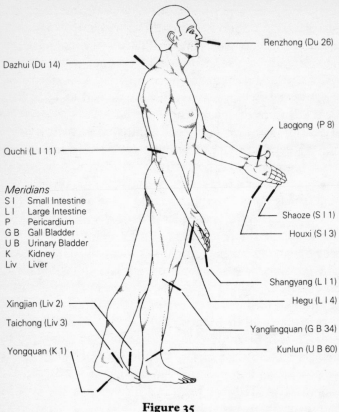

Figure 35

problem since it often occurs as a reaction to eating things like shellfish or strawberries. It may also occur as a result of emotional trauma. Its other name is nettle-rash, because the rash that it produces looks very similar to that which might occur on someone who has been badly stung by nettles.

If we picture a woman with urticaria, she has large raised red patches on her arms, legs, trunk and face. These appeared suddenly and are hot and itchy. On examination

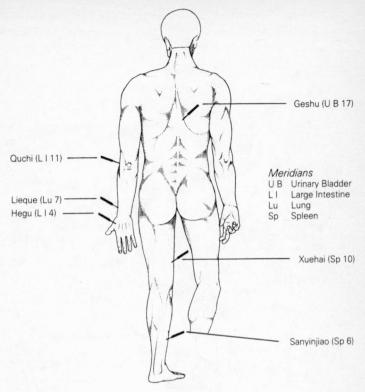

Geshu (U B 17)

Quchi (L I 11)

Meridians
U B   Urinary Bladder
L I   Large Intestine
Lu   Lung
Sp   Spleen

Lieque (Lu 7)
Hegu (L I 4)

Xuehai (Sp 10)

Sanyinjiao (Sp 6)

Figure 36

her tongue is red and has a thin yellow coating and her pulse is superficial in character and rapid. The redness of her skin patches, together with the red tongue and rapid pulse, suggest an invasion by heat, while the suddenness of onset and the yellow coating on the tongue indicate that wind is also involved. Thus treatment will be aimed at eliminating both of these factors. Figure 36 shows some of the points that may be used.

Heat is eliminated by using Xuehai, Sanyinjiao, Geshu ('diaphragm shu point'), Quchi and Hegu. The last two, and Lieque, also eliminate wind and, in addition, Hegu is a specific point for the treatment of skin conditions.

Nosebleeds

Some people are troubled by recurrent nosebleeds. Usually the bleeding occurs from an area at the back of the nose, known as Little's area, which is particularly well supplied with tiny blood vessels. These blood vessels may become fragile and bleed at the slightest provocation. If the nosebleeds become particularly frequent or severe, orthodox medicine offers cauterization of Little's area. This is a fairly minor procedure and usually stops further bleeding. Medication is also available which, if taken at the time of a nosebleed, will help to shut down these tiny blood vessels.

However, let us look at a patient who has not tried orthodox treatment and who has arrived at the acupuncture clinic just after having had a nosebleed. On examination he looks slightly flushed and his pulse is rapid. Haemorrhage is often due to invasion by heat. The nose is the sense organ that is associated with the lung so we can deduce from the patient's symptoms that there is an excess of heat in the Lung meridian, which is corroborated by the patient's pulse and his flushed appearance. Treatment consists of eradicating the heat.

Figure 37 shows some of the points that might be used. Hegu, Shaoshang ('young merchant') and Taixi all act to reduce heat in the lungs.

SOME CASE HISTORIES

Miss N. L.

Miss N. L. was a fifty-three-year-old woman who had suf-

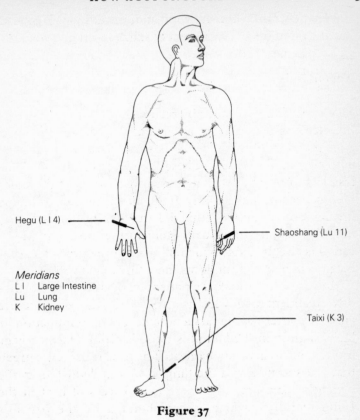

Hegu (L I 4)

Shaoshang (Lu 11)

Meridians
L I   Large Intestine
Lu   Lung
K   Kidney

Taixi (K 3)

Figure 37

fered from arthritis for a number of years. She was referred for acupuncture, reluctantly, by her general practitioner who would have preferred to send her to see the rheumatologist at the local hospital. However, Miss N. L. had had her fill of hospitals over the years and, having had some relief from her symptoms following a brief course of acupuncture five years previously, had decided to try it again.

Her story was that, at the age of ten, she was thrown from a horse and injured her back and shoulder. At the time, she seemed to make a full recovery and was soon riding again but, during her teens, she started to develop pain in her neck and shoulders. This continued to develop in her twenties and thirties. She saw an osteopath and the treatment he gave her produced temporary relief from pain. A few years later she saw a chiropractor, with a similar result. Finally, the only thing that resolved the pain for any length of time was injections into the painful areas. However, even these did not have a very lasting effect.

She had a brief course of acupuncture while visiting a friend in Scotland and felt, at the time, that, had she been able to continue, this might have been the answer to her problems. So when, a few years later, a friend told her that there was an acupuncturist within easy reach of her home, she decided to give it another try.

When she came for her first appointment, it was about a year since she had had the last course of injections and the pain had now returned and was worse than ever. She had been unable to sleep on her back for a number of years and she found that she could not stand to do housework for long periods of time. She cared for her elderly mother, who lived with her, as well as doing a part-time clerical job and was finding it increasingly difficult to cope. She suffered from recurrent sinusitis and was prone to chest infections which would result in her wheezing and coughing up large amounts of phlegm. She used an asthma inhaler regularly.

Over the years, the arthritis which had started in her back and shoulders – the areas injured by the fall from the horse – had spread, and she also felt pain in her knees and wrists and had developed a constant numb feeling in her left leg.

As I mentioned earlier, arthritis is said to be due to a blockage to the free flow of Chi, often due to initial injury. In this woman's case, the blockage seemed to involve mainly the Urinary Bladder and the Gall Bladder meridians and it appeared to be blockage of both of these, in their course down the leg, that was causing the numbness. On examination, she was very tender along the Gall Bladder meridian.

One method of unblocking a congested meridian is to treat points lying at the periphery of the involved area and thus encourage Chi to flow between them. The idea is that, gradually, the involved area will get smaller, the points being treated getting closer together, until finally Chi is flowing freely down the meridian.

In this woman's case, it was decided, first of all, to treat the peripheral points on the Gall Bladder meridian. It seemed as though this might have been the meridian that sustained the original damage and, sometimes, if one can treat the meridian that was affected by the initial injury, it is possible to resolve the problem without having to treat all the other meridians that have since become involved.

There is a sensation that occurs when acupuncture needles are inserted which is a good indication to the acupuncturist that 'something is happening' – in other words, that Chi is flowing. It is known by a variety of terms, such as needling sensation, or radiation, or the Chinese term 'deqi', and can take a number of forms. Usually the patient feels a tingling sensation or a numbness or, as some American acupuncturists describe it, a sensation of 'hurting good'. The one thing that this sensation should not be is unpleasantly painful. It is very hard to describe, but once a patient has experienced it, he will recognize it for what it is. Miss N. L. always experienced very clear radiation sensations and it was particularly interesting that, although she had no knowledge whatsoever of the theory of acupuncture, she was able to map out her meridians by describing the course that the radiation took.

At the first session of treatment, she had a good radiation sensation and the pain that she had been experiencing in her right shoulder quickly disappeared. After the session she felt very tired and developed a slight headache. However, that night, for the first time in ages, she was able to sleep comfortably on her back. The pain in her shoulder did not return but she was aware of severe pain in her back and her right leg. Although she had had a lifelong tendency to constipation, she started to have twice-daily bowel movements which she described as being 'as though the body was getting rid of poison'.

She came for her second session a week later. On this occasion, the peripheral points of both the Gall Bladder and the Urinary Bladder meridians were used. At the end of the session she was relatively pain free. Four days after the session, she experienced a brief period of pain which ran down the Gall Bladder meridian and she then developed a pain in her groin which she recalled that she had had a number of years previously. As in all alternative therapies, the recurrence of old symptoms is taken to be a good sign that the disease is regressing. One has to work backwards in time in order to rediscover the original healthy body, rather like peeling off layers of wallpaper that, over the years, have been stuck one on top of another in order, finally, to get to the underlying plastered wall.

At her next session, Miss N. L. told me that she had been to visit a friend and had found her in the middle of decorating her kitchen. Miss N. L. volunteered to help and spent two hours painting the ceiling. When she got home, she realized with some amazement that she had managed to do this without any pain developing in her shoulder.

On this occasion, the treatment given the previous week was repeated and, in addition, the source point of the Lung meridian was needled. This is the point that forms a direct link to the lung itself. It was used in view of Miss N. L.'s history of respiratory problems and because it was particularly tender, implying that it needed treating.

In the week following this session, Miss N. L. became

very much more mobile and described herself as being able to 'come downstairs like a puppy'. She also developed a cough and started to cough up large amounts of phlegm while, at the same time, her sinuses were draining profusely. Although she normally would have expected symptoms such as these to be accompanied by an attack of asthma, she had no wheezing whatsoever.

The treatment was repeated again and by the following session she had developed a pain in her back, just above her waist, which she remembered having about twenty years previously but not in the intervening years. Her chest was much better and movement was becoming a great deal easier.

Over the next two months she continued to attend weekly sessions and her condition improved steadily. Treatment remained pretty much the same with needling of the peripheral points of the disturbance. In addition, when she described the path taken by her radiation sensations, an extra needle would be inserted at the point to which the sensation ran, with other needles further up the meridian as the radiation was 'chased' up it. During this period she reported that she was feeling better with fewer asthma attacks and, as an added bonus, her eyesight had improved (this was actually confirmed by a trip to the optician).

Three months after Miss N. L. started treatment, a close friend of hers died and, for a month after this, her condition deteriorated slightly and did not respond to treatment.*

*I have not seen any mention of this phenomenon in the literature but I know that it has been observed by other acupuncturists of my acquaintance. I have also seen it myself in one other patient who failed to respond to treatment for a month following her father's death although, until then, she had been responding well. Why the period should be a month I do not know, but a colleague has suggested that it may be something to do with the lunar cycle. The early acupuncturists took into account not only the condition of the patient and the time of the day but also various astrological factors before they carried out treatment. Although this might seem a little far-fetched today, one has only to look at the science of biorhythms and, even more familiar, the monthly cycle of the average woman, to see that cyclical activity affects not just the solar system but also the human body.

After this month passed, Miss N. L. began to respond again to treatment and her arthritic pain, which had been considerable during this period, started to disappear again. The numbness, which had been worst around the region of her hip, was much reduced and seemed to be working its way down her leg. When describing the differences between internal and external diseases in Chapter Four, I mentioned the homoeopathic law known as Hering's Law of Cure, which states that things heal from the inside out and from the top down. Thus a pain, or in this case a sensation of numbness, which seems to be moving down the body is an indication of an improvement in the patient's condition.

Once the treatment started to work again, Miss N. L. found that she was going for a week at a time without having to use her asthma spray although it was the middle of winter, a time of year when normally she would have needed to use it every night.

Within the next three weeks, the pain became localized into the Urinary Bladder meridian and into the area which Miss N. L. had described as being that which sustained the original injury. Treatment continued using just the Urinary Bladder meridian, with needling of the peripheral points plus others that were specific for relieving congestion of Chi. The patient continued to make progress and reported the disappearance of the numbness in her leg, an absence of asthma despite the fact that she had caught a cold, and a further improvement in her eyesight. On one occasion she had some severe pain in her back as a result of a bout of over-enthusiastic gardening, but this improved following her next session.

After the first three months of treatment, she started to attend once a fortnight instead of weekly and, two months later, this was changed to one session every three weeks. After another two months, the treatments became monthly.

The pain became more and more localized, back into the area that had been injured when she was ten years old, before finally disappearing.

This woman's case illustrates that even long-standing problems may be helped by acupuncture, although it can take many months for them to resolve completely. However, as the acupuncturist is treating the energy flow in the whole patient, the patient can get some good 'fringe benefits' along the way as this woman did, with not just relief of her arthritis, but also an improvement in her asthmatic condition and in her eyesight.

Miss L. S.

Miss L. S. was a nurse who worked at the local general hospital. A major part of a nurse's work entails heavy lifting and it is not uncommon for them to suffer from back strain. Miss L. S. was used to lifting, but one day, after helping to lift a patient from a trolley into his bed on his return from the operating theatre, she developed severe pain in both shoulders, midway between the tip of the shoulder and the neck on each side. The pain lasted for several days during which time she was taking pain-killers at regular intervals, and it finally disappeared. Unfortunately, three weeks later, while lifting another patient, she experienced the pain again. And, again, it lasted for several days.

Miss L. S. now found that the pain would be brought back by lesser exertion than that which had caused it initially. Whenever it occurred, it would last for several days and she was unable to lift her arms without making the pain much worse. Finally, it started to interfere quite considerably with her work, despite the fact that she continued to take pain-killers, and she decided to seek help.

When she came for acupuncture, the pain had recurred

for the fifth time. She was not convinced that acupuncture would help but a friend had suggested it and, by this time, she was 'getting desperate'.

It seemed that the initial problem was a blockage to the flow of Chi, which had been caused by injury. On examination, the point at which she felt the pain on both sides was the site of the acupuncture point Jianjing ('well of the shoulder') and she was extremely tender over these points. A needle was inserted into Jianjing on each side and the pain rapidly resolved. At the end of the session the pain was only slight and had gone completely by the end of the day. Two years later it had still not recurred.

Mr B. V.

This twenty-four-year-old man woke up one morning to find that he was unable to move his right wrist. He could use his arm perfectly normally but his right hand hung limply and could not be raised. This sort of condition, known as wrist drop, is usually due to injury or prolonged pressure affecting the nerve supply to the muscles of the forearm and hand. However, in Mr B. V.'s case, no such history was forthcoming.

He was seen by the neurology specialist at the local hospital and a diagnosis of localized nerve damage was made. The only explanation seemed to be that Mr B. V. must have lain in such a position while asleep that somehow the nerve was stretched or damaged. Whatever the cause, though, the neurologist told him that there was no specific treatment and that he would just have to wait for the nerve to recover, something that could take between six months and two years. Meanwhile, he was to have physiotherapy which would prevent the affected muscles from contracting.

It was the physiotherapist who suggested that acupuncture might help and, accordingly, Mr B. V. attended for treatment. A sudden paralysis of this nature suggests an obstruction to the flow of Chi due to wind. Only points in the affected area, on the back of the hand, wrist and forearm, were used: Hegu to expel wind, Yanglao ('nourishment of the old') which is specific for local paralysis, Zhongshu ('central islet'), Yangchi and Waiguan, all of which unblock obstructions to the flow of Chi.

The patient was treated every other day for two weeks after which time he had recovered a considerable amount of movement in his wrist. He continued to have treatment twice a week and within six weeks he was back to normal.

Mr J. A.

Mr J. A. was a man of forty-three who, twenty years earlier, having taken a degree in geology at an English university, was offered a job with a large firm in Australia. He leapt at the chance of 'seeing the world' and undertook his new job with great enthusiasm. For a time, everything went very well. He was competent and well liked by the men with whom he worked. He met an Australian girl and they had plans to get married. However, one day there was a very serious accident at the site at which he was working and two men were badly mutilated.

It was Mr J. A.'s job to write out the reports of these accidents and it was while doing so that his right arm suddenly stopped functioning. He could grip the pen with his hand but was quite unable to move his arm. He saw the company doctor who could not explain what had happened and suggested that it might be some localized form of polio. After several weeks there was no sign of recovery and, eventually, Mr J. A. lost his job on the grounds of chronic incapacity. He was thoroughly depressed by this and even more so by the fact that no one could tell him what had caused the problem or whether it was ever likely to get better. He was unable to face looking for another job in a country that was not his home and so, breaking off his engagement, he left for England.

Back home, he found it hard to get a job and had to take whatever he could get. But he remained unsettled, his arm was not improving and the muscles were beginning to waste. After a succession of jobs which offered him no mental challenge, he decided to start his own business. It was around this time, too, that he met an English girl and married her.

Unfortunately, he was dogged by bad luck and, eventually, his business capsized and he was left with serious financial problems. He struggled on but was having difficulties at home as well. He and his wife were not getting on and finally they divorced. He found a job but, as before, it was no challenge to him and this, together with his divorce and his financial problems, produced a severe depression and he became suicidal.

At the height of these problems, he decided to have some acupuncture treatment on the recommendation of a friend. The acupuncturist who treated him is a practitioner of the Five Elements school. He diagnosed that the patient had an imbalance in his Earth meridians. This was based on the fact that his face appeared to have yellow lines, his voice was singing in character and he craved sympathy. In addition, the acupuncturist was impressed by the patient's great interest in geology and things of the earth. The Earth meridians are those of the Spleen and the Stomach and, on taking Mr J. A.'s pulses, the two corresponding to these meridians were found to be bounding.

The treatment comprised sedation of the meridians that were in excess, together with transfer of energy from them to weaker meridians by the use of specific transfer points.

In addition, the source points of the Stomach and Spleen meridians were used as these are the direct links to the stomach and spleen themselves. The element points – that is, the Earth points – on both meridians were also used.

After two months of treatment, although there was, as yet, no noticeable difference in his arm, the patient's whole attitude to life started to change. The depression left him and he started to think in a far more positive manner than before. He began to talk about returning to Australia and seeing if he could find his fiancée of twenty years before. After four months he started to regain some movement in his arm and was referred by his general practitioner to the local hospital for physiotherapy.

After nine months of treatment, Mr J. A. returned to Australia. Two months later his acupuncturist received a letter to say that he had met up again with his first fiancée. She had married a year after he had left Australia but the marriage had not lasted. They were now intending to get married shortly and make up for lost time. His arm, he said, was continuing to improve and he was hoping to find an acupuncturist in Adelaide where they were settling, so that he could continue treatment.

Mr D. K.

This forty-five-year-old man rang up the acupuncturist one Friday afternoon asking for an emergency appointment. He had severe toothache and needed some treatment to control it until he could see the dentist on the Monday morning.

His history was an interesting one. He had been a high-powered executive in a large company for a number of years and the pressures under which he worked were enormous. His sphere of responsibility gradually grew until, to relieve the stress, he started to drink. His alcohol intake increased until he was drinking a bottle of whisky or more a day. By this time, it was the alcohol that was making it impossible for him to cope with his job and he was replaced.

After this trauma, he found himself another job and managed to stop drinking with the aid of Alcoholics Anonymous, but his body began to react to all the various stresses that he had been under and he started to develop allergies. At first, these were allergies to common allergens such as pollen and cats' fur; then he started to find that certain foods would make him vomit; finally substances such as diesel fumes began to affect him so that he was unable to walk along a busy road without feeling sick and faint.

He went to see a specialist at the local hospital and was started on a course of desensitizing injections. He was warned that this would be a long job, since there were so many things that he seemed to be allergic to. When he developed toothache, he knew that he would be unable to visit the dentist immediately, as he would have been affected by the anaesthetic gases present in the air which had accumulated during the week. The only answer was to get an appointment for first thing on Monday morning when, after the weekend, the surgery would be relatively free of gas. Meanwhile, he wanted some acupuncture to control the pain.

Now, acupuncture can be used for emergency treatment but it is best used to give a course of treatment. The reason for this is that, when one is manipulating energies, although temporary relief can be obtained from one treatment, problems may occur at a later date if the energies are not completely returned to normal. So when Mr D. K. phoned for an emergency acupuncture appointment, he was told that he would only be treated if he agreed to come for a follow-up course of treatment.

Accordingly, Mr D. K. came and his toothache was treated by the insertion of two needles. The pain was relieved for thirty-six hours and, on the Monday morning, he went to see the dentist. When he returned to see the acupuncturist, a diagnosis was made according to the Law of the Five Elements. The element which seemed to be out of balance in his case was metal. This was a case of deficiency and the signs on which the acupuncturist based his diagnosis showed problems with both metal and water. Water is the child of metal, so that deficiency in the mother can produce an undernourished child – the so-called screaming child syndrome. In Mr D. K.'s case, he showed grief and anguish when he talked about his problems and his voice had a weeping quality, which indicated metal. However, his face had a bluish look to it and his bodily smell seemed putrid, signifying the involvement of water.

The treatment consisted of stimulating the deficient metal, using primarily the element points (that is, the Metal points on the Metal meridians, Large Intestine and Lung) and also the source points on the Metal meridians.

After his fourth session of treatment, an improvement was noticeable and Mr D. K. spoke to the consultant at the hospital about the necessity of continuing with the injections. As a result, these were gradually reduced. After four months of acupuncture treatment, he had stopped the injections and all trace of the allergies had disappeared.

Mr P. S.

Mr P. S. was a thirty-two-year-old policeman who had joined the force some eight years earlier, after coming out of the Army. Although he enjoyed his job, he found it stressful and for the past three years had been taking tranquillizers regularly.

He had coped with a number of fairly traumatic incidents in his earlier life, including a very severe accident at the age of twenty-one, when he had been knocked off his motor cycle. He had been in Intensive Care for three months following this but had ultimately made a full recovery and had been able to return to his Army duties. When he was twenty-five he had been posted to Northern Ireland for two years and, during the time he was there, had twice narrowly escaped being killed and had seen a friend badly injured.

All this stress had taken its toll and he had become a chain-smoker. And although his job in the police force was far less stressful than what he had previously been through, he had much less resistance than before. He had recurrent symptoms of severe chest pain and severe back pain, accompanied by shivering. On two occasions, he had been rushed to hospital with a presumed diagnosis of a heart attack. The tranquillizers did not seem to reduce his symptoms but he was scared of doing without them, in case things got even worse. He described himself as being full of fear.

He had got to the stage where he could see that, sooner or later, he would not be able to carry on with his job, so he decided to look for help and, on the advice of a colleague, made an appointment for some acupuncture, with the idea of trying to get rid of the chest pain.

He was diagnosed, according to the Law of the Five Elements, as having problems relating to metal. This was based on the weeping quality of his voice, the anguish and grief with which he told his story, the white appearance of his face and his putrid bodily smell. However, the acupuncturist decided that he was also suffering from a complete obstruction to the circulation of Chi. He therefore started treatment using a combination of needles which is known as the Treatment of the Seven Dragons. This is used specifically in cases where there is a severe disruption of energy flow affecting the whole body, and it is interesting to note that the position of several of the needles used in this correspond to the positions of the major chakras, which are said by healers to be the major energy centres of the body. (Healing, like acupuncture, is based on the idea of manipulating energies.) After the treatment, Mr P. S. started to tremble. This became quite severe and continued for about forty-five minutes after the needles had been removed, after which time it started to subside.

Follow-up treatments consisted of strengthening the heart and the Heart meridian, since the heart is associated with fire, and metal is the servant of fire, so that weakness of fire can result in it losing control of metal. The Metal source points and element points were also used.

After only a few treatments, the patient was able to stop taking his tranquillizers and, after several months, had lost all his anxiety and was enjoying life to the full.

CHAPTER EIGHT

ACUPUNCTURE AND

MODERN SCIENCE

We live today in a scientific and materialistic world in which miracles don't happen – or, if they do, they must be explained or disproved. In the last few decades, science has developed to such an extent that everything now has to be proved scientifically in order to be acceptable. All too often science has made it impossible for us to accept something which cannot be readily explained in its own terms, and charlatans and forgers over the years have helped to make sceptics of us all. Complementary medicine has suffered greatly in this respect. To those who have been brought up in the West, in an environment of hospitals and health services, doctors and dentists, the complementary therapies, particularly some of the rather more 'way out' ones, seem to be in much the same category as spiritualism and fortune-telling.

One of the main stumbling blocks that has prevented a wider acceptance of the complementary therapies is the fact that they use a completely different vocabulary from orthodox medicine and science. The terms in which acupuncture is explained, the concept of Chi and of the meridians, are not easily assimilated into Western thinking. To suggest to a Western-trained scientist that acupuncture works by the manipulation of, to him, unproven body energies is as convincing as saying that a conjuring trick works because the magician says 'abracadabra'. In short, acupuncture is 'unscientific'. But many Western physicians are aware that acupuncture works and are interested in using it. However, although they can accept the fact that the therapy is of value, they are unable to accept the terms in which it is explained. And so these physicians and scientists, wishing to use acupuncture but not understanding it, have felt obliged to 'explain' its workings and to interpret it into their own terminology and concepts.

There is, of course, nothing intrinsically wrong in this. If you wish a Frenchman who only knows his mother tongue to appreciate a book that has been written in English you must translate it into French. This is perfectly acceptable. When it starts to become a problem is when the Frenchman declares that until the works of Shakespeare, Jane Austen and Chaucer have been translated into French, they are of no value. It is quite understandable that Western physicians should wish to know how acupuncture works in their own terms – that is, related to the nervous system and physiology as they know it. However, there are those who maintain that until such time as it has been proved scientifically to them that certain nervous reflexes are involved in acupuncture and that the results achieved are all scientifically 'above board', they will regard acupuncture as suspect.

Anyone who has taken the time to look at acupuncture will tell you there is no doubt that it works. And patients, who have been treated with acupuncture and, as a result, have recovered from illnesses which orthodox practitioners had told them they must learn to live with, will tell you that they don't care how it works. Acupuncture has shown, over a period of two thousand years and more, that it works. Scientific investigation of its workings should not be deemed essential in order to corroborate that fact.

It has to be said that Western physicians still do not fully understand the nervous system, which is the most complex system of the body. So experiments demonstrating pseudo-acupuncture effects are only showing those effects in the light of an incompletely understood system. It is as though we had discovered that our Frenchman understood a little German and, instead of translating the great works of English literature into French for him, we translated them into German. He will probably understand the gist of the stories, but to get the full meaning he will have to use a dictionary and spend many more hours studying the language.

Of course, in none of these scientific experiments is any attention paid to the concept of the life force. This doesn't come into physiology at all. While we are building bigger and better machines and computers which become more and more like man, able to take over his work and perhaps to do it even better than he does, we are also reducing man himself to the level of a machine. However, there comes a point at which both tendencies, the building up of the machines and the reduction of man, reach an impasse from which they cannot escape, simply because there will always be the difference – that a live man or woman is permeated by a life force; when that force goes, the body dies. A machine has no such force and therefore can be repaired almost *ad infinitum*, providing that replacement parts are always available. You can carry on replacing parts of a machine until there is nothing of the original machine left – yet, fundamentally, it is still the same machine. You cannot do that with a living being.

Such a concept does seem to take us into the realms of theology, since the life force could be compared to what theologians would call spirit. Much science fiction has been written about the creation of living beings by man. But, although it is possible to manufacture protein and the other components of man in a test tube, no one has found out how to create a living thing from first principles. The life force remains elusive.

The idea of the merging of disciplines, of the transition between chemistry and biology, between botany and zoology, even between theology and science, takes us back

to the idea of holism, which is the basis of so many complementary therapies. A colleague of mine observed that many
Western practitioners are valiantly trying to adopt the concept of holism, but to them it still means looking at the
patient as a whole – but divided into body, mind and spirit –
whereas, of course, true holism entails just looking at the
patient. Body, mind and spirit form a whole and, just
because the former can be more fully explained than the
other two, and the last can be explained not at all, they cannot be divided from each other.

Having said all that, we will do no harm by asking how
acupuncture is related to physiology as understood by
Western physicians. Many of the experiments that demonstrate the workings of the nervous system are performed on
animals (a highly controversial issue in itself). These have
shown us that stimulation of certain points on the skin can
produce effects at a distance from these points which seem
to be dependent on the normal functioning of the nervous
system. Because animal experimentation permits the de-
struction of various parts of the animal's nervous system,
we also have been able to find out which part of the nervous
system carries the signal. What is interesting is that in the
nervous system theory of acupuncture, depending on
which part of the body is stimulated, the nervous impulses
that seem to be responsible for producing the effect appear
to be carried in different ways. It is difficult, therefore, to
propound an overall theory explaining, in Western terms,
how acupuncture works.

For example, experiments have been performed in which
stimulation of the skin on the back of rats produced changes
in their intestines. The results were found to be the same
whether the rat's nervous system was intact or whether the
spinal cord had been divided, thus cutting off the body
from the brain. From this it was deduced that the nervous
impulses controlling the effects of stimulation were entirely

confined to the spinal cord. However, a similar experiment performed on fish, where stimulation of the lower part of the bowel produced changes in the skin, was found to be effective even if the spinal cord had been destroyed. In this case, another section of the nervous system, the sympathetic nervous system, seemed to be involved in producing the result.

Felix Mann, in his book *Acupuncture: the Ancient Chinese Art of Healing*, puts forward a theory that the responses obtained in various organs of the body when points on the skin are stimulated tie in with the way in which the body develops as an embryo. Each section of the body, together with its nerve supply, develops from a different section of the embryo. Physicians call these sections dermatomes. Very often, both an organ and the acupuncture points that affect it lie in the same dermatome. However, Felix Mann points out that the 'acupuncture points of the legs and head do not fit in with what is known of dermatomes'. This means that another theory has to be found to explain how acupuncture works in these parts of the body.

While the medical profession struggles to understand how acupuncture works, acupuncture anaesthesia has become quite respectable, thanks to the discovery of endorphins.

Endorphins are naturally occurring substances which are released from the body to produce a pain-killing effect. It would appear that individuals differ in their normal levels of endorphins, circulating in the blood stream. This may explain why different people have different pain thresholds, some being able to tolerate far more pain than others. Secretion of large amounts of endorphins occurs in response to severe pain, for example during childbirth and after injury.

Stimulation of acupuncture points that produce anaesthetic effects has been shown to release endorphins into the body. What has not been explained, at least in Western terms, is why stimulation of these particular points and no others produces these effects.

A colleague of mine once said that the discovery of endorphins was the best thing that had happened to acupuncture because it enabled the medical profession to accept the validity of acupuncture. 'Western thought', she said, 'has got this wonderful ability to say that if you can't explain it, it doesn't exist.' This attitude is rather odd when you consider that, as far as I am aware, no one has yet explained fully the way in which aspirin works, nor some of the antidepressants, nor many of the drugs that are handed out, day after day, in the general practitioner's surgery. On the whole, the basic biochemical action of such drugs is understood, that is, how it reacts in the body and what the effects of those reactions are. But, in many cases, the way in which those chemical reactions produce the final effects felt by the patient is poorly understood. The medical profession, nevertheless, is satisfied that the drug produces the same effect time and time again and therefore it is used for that purpose. When it comes to acupuncture, however, the fact that certain treatments can produce certain results time and time again is disregarded because 'we don't know how it works'.

Of course, this attitude is not representative of the entire medical profession. Many of its members are now becoming very interested in complementary therapies and are coming round to the view that 'if it works and is safe, then it should be used, even if we don't fully understand how it works'. It is, indeed, very difficult for an orthodox practitioner, brought up in the realms of things that he can see and measure – nerves producing electrical impulses, red blood cells carrying oxygen, kidney cells secreting waste products into the urine – to accept things that cannot be seen or measured, but just have to be taken on trust.

In one way, it is easier to accept acupuncture than it is to accept some of the other therapies. The acupuncture meridians can be seen as the ancient Chinese description of the nervous system and the effects of acupuncture may, to a certain extent, be explained as functions of the nervous system. The theories on which healing, radionics and homoeopathy are founded are much harder for an orthodox physician to understand. However, practitioners of these systems would find it relatively easy to accept the philosophy of acupuncture. In healing and radionics, for example, energy is said to flow through a system of nadis – a fine network of channels that pervades and surrounds the entire body. Thus it is easy for a healer to understand the system of meridians as an aspect of the nadis and for the acupuncturist to understand the nadis as an extension of the meridians. So, in the end, it may well be acupuncture which acts as a bridge to bring together the practitioners of orthodox and unorthodox therapies by having a component that both sides can understand or relate to.

Attitudes are changing and more and more orthodox practitioners are referring patients to acupuncturists and are even using acupuncture themselves (I shall say more about this in the following chapter). It is an important step forward. For, as a colleague once said, 'If we all stood around waiting for things to be fully explained before we used them, we'd still be watching television by candle-light!'

CHAPTER NINE

FINDING OUT

ABOUT TREATMENT

Now that acupuncture has become popular in the West, training schools are being established so that aspiring acupuncturists no longer have to travel to China in order to learn how to use the therapy. This means that there are an increasing number of acupuncturists working in the West, some of whom are doctors and some of whom practise, in addition, other alternative therapies. There is, as yet, no overall governing body which regulates the training and practice of acupuncturists in the same way that the General Medical Council is in charge of the training and conduct of doctors in the United Kingdom. The various colleges teach in different ways and award their own qualifications. And there are numerous short courses available, especially for doctors, which offer no qualifications as such. Two of the main colleges in the United Kingdom are the College of Traditional Chinese Acupuncture in Leamington Spa, Warwickshire, which teaches the Five Elements system of acupuncture, and the International College of Oriental Medicine in East Grinstead, Sussex, which teaches the Eight Syndromes system. According to the length of time they have studied acupuncture, graduates of the College of Traditional Chinese Acupuncture may put the letters Lic. Ac., B. Ac., M. Ac. or D. Ac. after their names. Graduates of the International College of Oriental Medicine may become B. Ac., M. Ac. or D. Ac. There are other colleges, such as the British College of Acupuncture, which teach acupuncture from a Western viewpoint and these, too, award L. Ac., B. Ac. and D. Ac. qualifications. There is also the Liu Clinic in Gunnersbury, London, which awards no such qualifications but teaches traditional Chinese medicine and acupuncture and gives its own diplomas.

So, whom does one go to for treatment? It might, on the whole, be easier to say whom one should not go to. As a rule of thumb, for any of the alternative therapies, one should avoid practitioners who advertise. This is because the majority of governing bodies in the world of alternative therapies, like the General Medical Council, forbid practitioners who are registered with them to advertise. Therefore, if a practitioner advertises, it is often an indication that he is not fully trained and registered. However, this does not apply to a listing in the Yellow Pages telephone directory (even doctors are allowed to be in this) nor, in some cases such as registered homoeopaths, to 'announcements'. The latter encompasses a single announcement in a newspaper to the effect that the practitioner is available to see patients. It does not include regular advertisements on the lines of: 'Do you have backache? Migraine? Arthritis? Acupuncture therapy will help. Ring Joe Bloggs'.

Of course, one very good way of finding a practitioner is to ask around among your friends. A personal recommendation is well worth having. If the condition that you want treated is a fairly straightforward one involving the bones or muscles, such as arthritis, there is no reason why it should not be adequately treated by a doctor who has done a short course of acupuncture. Your general practitioner may well know of someone to whom he can refer you. However, many doctors who now practise acupuncture have only done short courses and they use the treatment symptomatically – in other words, they are not concerned with the holistic application of balancing the patient's energies but only with alleviating his symptoms (usually pain). This may be all right if all you need is pain relief. In fact, many of the doctors who practise acupuncture are anaesthetists and rheumatologists who use it in their pain clinics. Doctors, too, are just as good at putting in ear studs to help smokers and weight-watchers as anybody else.

However, if your problem is a more complicated one or if you feel that you need the holistic approach, try to make sure that your acupuncturist is one who uses either the system of the Five Elements or the system of the Eight Syndromes. If you ring an acupuncturist with a view to going for treatment, it is quite permissible to ask him what form of treatment he uses. Tell him your problem, briefly, and ask whether he thinks he can help. Sometimes, it is an advantage to go to a therapist who is working in a natural therapies centre since, if the acupuncturist does not think he can help you, he may be able to refer you to a colleague whose therapy he thinks may suit you better, such as herbalism, homoeopathy or osteopathy. Sometimes an acupuncturist may also practise other therapies and this can be beneficial. There is no doubt that two therapies together may sometimes work better than one alone and, in my experience, the effects of acupuncture may be increased when used together with manipulation or with healing.

Graduates of the College of Traditional Chinese Acupuncture become members of the Traditional Acupuncture Society and appear on its register. Graduates of the International College of Oriental Medicine appear on the Register of Traditional Chinese Medicine. Practitioners who appear on the register of the British Acupuncture Association have all passed the examinations set by the British College of Acupuncture. These organizations, which have a common code of ethics, are now liaising on the Council for Acupuncture which is trying to agree standards for acupuncture training in Britain. The Institute for Complementary Medicine can put prospective patients in touch with qualified therapists in many fields of complementary medicine. The addresses of these organizations, together with those of the acupuncture colleges, are given at the end of this book. One does not need a doctor's letter to see an acupuncturist, unless the latter happens to be a doctor himself. However, it is often advisable to inform your general practitioner that you intend to have some acupuncture therapy, for many a sceptical doctor has been convinced as to the value of a complementary therapy after seeing one of his patients make a (to him) unexpected recovery.

Of course, like all therapies, acupuncture does not work for everybody. However, if you go to a reputable practitioner, you can be sure that he will not keep bringing you back if you are unlikely to respond. Depending on how long you have been ill, it may take a while before you begin to respond, so you must be patient, but the practitioner ought to be able to tell you at what stage you should start thinking about trying another therapy if nothing seems to be happening. Some practitioners ask patients to commit themselves to six, or even twelve, sessions in order to give the therapy a good chance of working. Usually, if one is going to get results, there will be some improvement in the patient's condition by the fourth or fifth treatment. Once you do start to improve, it is very important to keep on with the treatment until the acupuncturist says you can stop. This goes back to the business of balancing energies. Energies have to flow and the first few treatments will start them flowing again but, if treatment is not continued, they can easily flow back to how they were before, leaving the patient just as unbalanced, but perhaps with different symptoms.

Treatment can take a long time (homoeopaths state that in order to return a patient completely to normal, they will need to treat him, on average, for one month for every year that he has been ill). Therefore, it can be expensive. If there appear to be several equally well-qualified acupuncturists local to you, there is no harm in asking what they charge before making an appointment. You may be surprised at the difference in prices. As far as ear studs are concerned, I have heard of two acupuncturists working within twenty miles of each other, with one charging over ten times as much as the other for the insertion of an ear stud. And, if it's an ear stud that you want, enquire whether the acupuncturist does regular checks. They do need to be changed every two weeks, so avoid a practitioner who doesn't do this.

And now, having made your appointment, what can you expect when you go for treatment? Well, of course, the acupuncturist will want to know your full history, that is, how long you have had the illness and information about your past medical history. He will also examine your tongue, pulse, skin and nails, depending on what system of diagnosis he uses. And he will then make you comfortable on a couch or chair, and insert the relevant needles.

Many people have become alarmed in recent times about the possibility of catching infections from unsterilized needles and, for this reason, prefer to see a doctor rather than a lay acupuncturist. However, lay acupuncturists have to be registered with their local councils who are responsible for inspecting the premises and the sterilizing equipment used. If this has been done, a certificate of inspection should be displayed in the clinic. In fact, all acupuncturists who have been trained at one of the recognized colleges will have been taught all about the necessity for sterilizing needles and, in many cases, will have more sophisticated sterilizing equipment than that normally found in a doctor's surgery! A number of practitioners now use pre-sterilized disposable needles.

As the needles go in, you are likely to feel the radiation, or needling, sensation that I mentioned in Chapter Seven. This can sometimes be quite fierce and may radiate a fairly long way. Sometimes patients feel slightly sick at this point, but this only lasts a second or two. Some patients experience a warm glow travelling along the length of the meridian and, occasionally, this is accompanied by a flush on the skin. It is important to keep as still as possible while the needles are in, in order to avoid dislodging them.

After the treatment the patient may feel considerably better. However, it is vital he remembers that he is not yet better. I have had several patients who, despite warnings, have been so delighted at being relatively free from pain that they have done more physical work in the house or in the garden than they should have and have set themselves back again. Having acupuncture treatment is like having a broken leg put into plaster. Once the plaster has set, the leg is comfortable and it is possible, if one is careful, to walk with the aid of a stick. However, the leg is still broken inside its plaster cast and needs to be allowed to rest in order to heal properly. In the same way, the initial acupuncture treatments will only start the energy flowing again, if the patient has been ill for some time. They will not heal him straight away and he must be patient and work with the treatment, no matter how exciting may be the prospect of doing things that he was previously unable to do.

Occasionally, after a session of acupuncture, the patient's symptoms may become a great deal worse. This, surprisingly, is a good sign. It also occurs in other therapies, such as homoeopathy where it is known as aggravation, and in healing where it is called a healing reaction. It is always a sign that the patient is going to respond well to treatment, and should be an encouragement to continue with treatment rather than an indication to give it up. The reaction usually lasts twenty-four hours or less and is often followed fairly quickly by a considerable improvement in the condition.

One thing that people are always aware of when they go to see an alternative practitioner is that he has far more time to give them than the average general practitioner, who is usually rushing to get through a waiting room full of patients in order to get out to see a list of bed-ridden patients in order to get back to do the next surgery – and so on, *ad infinitum*. A visit to an alternative practitioner is far more leisurely and there is greater opportunity for asking questions about one's condition and the treatment being given. Some practitioners will do home visits for patients whose condition prevents them getting to the surgery, and this is something else that you can ask about when you first contact an acupuncturist.

At present there is little use of acupuncture in place of anaesthesia, except in the Far East. However, since a number of anaesthetists use acupuncture in their pain clinics, it is possible that some might be willing to use it for suitable patients having minor operations. It is certainly possible to have acupuncture instead of pain-killers during childbirth and this has the great advantage that there is no risk to the baby. For a mother who is having a home confinement, arrangements can be made with an acupuncturist of her choice and with the midwife who is to do the delivery. In the case of a hospital confinement, however, it will be the obstetric consultant who will have to give his permission for an acupuncturist to treat the patient while she is in the labour ward.

One great advantage of acupuncture and the other holistic therapies is that, fairly early on in the treatment, the patient is likely to start feeling better – possibly even before the symptoms of his disease start to improve (a case in point was Mr J. A. who was mentioned in Chapter Seven). The ultimate aim of acupuncture is to bring the patient into perfect balance, for it is this balance, and not just an absence of disease, that constitutes good health.

USEFUL ADDRESSES

Training colleges

British College of Acupuncture, 44 New Market Square, Basingstoke, Hampshire (0256 46533).

College of Traditional Chinese Acupuncture, Tao House, Queensway, Leamington Spa, Warwickshire CM23 EZ (0926 22121).

International College of Oriental Medicine, Green Hedges House, Green Hedges Avenue, East Grinstead, W. Sussex RH19 1DZ (0342 28567).

Liu Clinic of Traditional Chinese Medicine, 13 Gunnersbury Avenue, London W5 3XD (01 993 2549/01 992 2611).

Organizations providing lists of qualified acupuncturists

British Acupuncture Association, 34 Alderney Street, London SW1V 4EU (01 834 3353/1012).

Council for Acupuncture, Suite 1, 19A Cavendish Square, London W1M 9AD (01 409 1440).

Council for Complementary and Alternative Medicine, Suite 1, 19A Cavendish Square, London W1M 9AD (01 409 1440).

Institute for Complementary Medicine, 21 Portland Place, London W1N 3AF (01 636 9543).

Register of Traditional Chinese Medicine, 18 Shenley Road, London SE5 (01 701 7107).

Traditional Acupuncture Society, 11 Grange Park, Stratford upon Avon, Warwickshire, CV37 6XH (0789 292507).

INDEX

FOR THE BEST IN PAPERBACKS, LOOK FOR THE

In every corner of the world, on every subject under the sun, Penguins represent quality and variety – the very best in publishing today.

For complete information about books available from Penguin and how to order them, write to us at the appropriate address below. Please note that for copyright reasons the selection of books varies from country to country.

In the United Kingdom: For a complete list of books available from Penguin in the U.K., please write to *Dept EP, Penguin Books Ltd, Harmondsworth, Middlesex, UB7 0DA*

In the United States: For a complete list of books available from Penguin in the U.S., please write to *Dept BA, Viking Penguin, 299 Murray Hill Parkway, East Rutherford, New Jersey 07073*

In Canada: For a complete list of books available from Penguin in Canada, please write to *Penguin Books Canada Limited, 2801 John Street, Markham, Ontario L3R 1B4*

In Australia: For a complete list of books available from Penguin in Australia, please write to the *Marketing Department, Penguin Books Australia Ltd, P.O. Box 257, Ringwood, Victoria 3134*

In New Zealand: For a complete list of books available from Penguin in New Zealand, please write to the *Marketing Department, Penguin Books (N.Z.) Ltd, Private Bag, Takapuna, Auckland 9*

In India: For a complete list of books available from Penguin in India, please write to *Penguin Overseas Ltd, 706 Eros Apartments, 56 Nehru Place, New Delhi 110019*

FOR THE BEST IN PAPERBACKS, LOOK FOR THE 🐧

COOKERY IN PENGUINS

Jane Grigson's Vegetable Book   Jane Grigson

The ideal guide to the cooking of everything from artichoke to yams, written with her usual charm and depth of knowledge by 'the most engaging food writer to emerge during the last few years' – *The Times*

More Easy Cooking for One or Two   Louise Davies

This charming book, full of ideas and easy recipes, offers even the novice cook good wholesome food with the minimum of effort.

The Cuisine of the Rose   Mireille Johnston

Classic French cooking from Burgundy and Lyonnais, including the most succulent dishes of meat and fish bathed in pungent sauces of wine and herbs.

Good Food from Your Freezer   Helge Rubinstein and Sheila Bush

Using a freezer saves endless time and trouble and cuts your food bills dramatically; this book will enable you to cook just as well – perhaps even better – with a freezer as without.

An Invitation to Indian Cooking   Madhur Jaffrey

A witty, practical and delightful handbook of Indian cookery by the much loved presenter of the successful television series.

Budget Gourmet   Geraldene Holt

Plan carefully, shop wisely and cook well to produce first-rate food at minimal expense. It's as easy as pie!

Mediterranean Food   Elizabeth David

Based on a collection of recipes made when the author lived in France, Italy, the Greek Islands and Egypt, this was the first book by Britain's greatest cookery writer.

The Complete Barbecue Book   James Marks

Mouth-watering recipes and advice on all aspects of barbecuing make this an ideal and inspired guide to *al fresco* entertainment.

A Book of Latin American Cooking   Elisabeth Lambert Ortiz

Anyone who thinks Latin American food offers nothing but *tacos* and *tortillas* will enjoy the subtle marriages of texture and flavour celebrated in this marvellous guide to one of the world's most colourful *cuisines*.

Quick Cook   Beryl Downing

For victims of the twentieth century, this book provides some astonishing gourmet meals – all cooked in under thirty minutes.

Josceline Dimbleby's Book of Puddings, Desserts and Savouries

'Full of the most delicious and novel ideas for every type of pudding' – *Lady*

Chinese Food   Kenneth Lo

A popular step-by-step guide to the whole range of delights offered by Chinese cookery and the fascinating philosophy behind it.

Audrey Eyton's F-Plus   Audrey Eyton

'Your short-cut to the most sensational diet of the century' – *Daily Express*

Caring Well for an Older Person   Muir Gray and Heather McKenzie

Wide-ranging and practical, with a list of useful addresses and contacts, this book will prove invaluable for anyone professionally concerned with the elderly or with an elderly relative to care for.

Baby and Child   Penelope Leach

A beautifully illustrated and comprehensive handbook on the first five years of life. 'It stands head and shoulders above anything else available at the moment' – Mary Kenny in the *Spectator*

Woman's Experience of Sex   Sheila Kitzinger

Fully illustrated with photographs and line drawings, this book explores the riches of women's sexuality at every stage of life. 'A book which any mother could confidently pass on to her daughter – and her partner too' – *Sunday Times*

Food Additives   Erik Millstone

Eat, drink and be worried? Erik Millstone's hard-hitting book contains powerful evidence about the massive risks being taken with the health of consumers. It takes the lid off the food we eat and takes the lid off the food industry.

Pregnancy and Diet   Rachel Holme

It *is* possible to eat well and healthily when pregnant while avoiding excessive calories; this book, with suggested foods, a sample diet-plan of menus and advice on nutrition, shows how.

Medicines: A Guide for Everybody   Peter Parish

This fifth edition of a comprehensive survey of all the medicines available over the counter or on prescription offers clear guidance for the ordinary reader as well as invaluable information for those involved in health care.

Pregnancy and Childbirth   Sheila Kitzinger

A complete and up-to-date guide to physical and emotional preparation for pregnancy – a must for all prospective parents.

The Penguin Encyclopaedia of Nutrition   John Yudkin

This book cuts through all the myths about food and diets to present the real facts clearly and simply. 'Everyone should buy one' – *Nutrition News and Notes*

The Parents' A to Z   Penelope Leach

For anyone with a child of 6 months, 6 years or 16 years, this guide to all the little problems involved in their health, growth and happiness will prove reassuring and helpful.

Jane Fonda's Workout Book

Help yourself to better looks, superb fitness and a whole new approach to health and beauty with this world-famous and fully illustrated programme of diet and exercise advice.

Alternative Medicine   Andrew Stanway

Dr Stanway provides an objective and practical guide to thirty-two alternative forms of therapy – from Acupuncture and the Alexander Technique to Macrobiotics and Yoga.

PENGUIN HEALTH

A Complete Guide to Therapy   Joel Kovel

The options open to anyone seeking psychiatric help are both numerous and confusing. Dr Kovel cuts through the many myths and misunderstandings surrounding today's therapy and explores the pros and cons of various types of therapies.

Pregnancy   Dr Jonathan Scher and Carol Dix

Containing the most up-to-date information on pregnancy – the effects of stress, sexual intercourse, drugs, diet, late maternity and genetic disorders – this book is an invaluable and reassuring guide for prospective parents.

Yoga   Ernest Wood

'It has been asked whether in yoga there is something for everybody. The answer is "yes"'   Ernest Wood.

Depression   Ross Mitchell

Depression is one of the most common contemporary problems. But what exactly do we mean by the term? In this invaluable book Ross Mitchell looks at depression as a mood, as an experience, as an attitude to life and as an illness.

Vogue Natural Health and Beauty   Bronwen Meredith

Health foods, yoga, spas, recipes, natural remedies and beauty preparations are all included in this superb, fully illustrated guide and companion to the bestselling *Vogue Body and Beauty Book*.

Care of the Dying   Richard Lamerton

It is never true that 'nothing more can be done' for the dying. This book shows us how to face death without pain, with humanity, with dignity and in peace.